Beyond Self-Esteem

Discovering Your Boundless Self-Worth

By Eloisa Ramos,
EFT Master,
Certified EFT Expert II

www.healing-with-eft.com

Cover design, formatting, editing and uploading by **Diego Ramos**. For eBook creation services contact me at: **Writingfiction.co@gmail.com, or Ramosink.com@gmail.com**

ISBN: 978-1-62154-078-6 (eBook)

ISBN: 9-781477-479223 (Paperback)

ACKNOWLEDGMENTS

This book is a personal perspective based on my experience and insights received in working with EFT (Emotional Freedom Techniques) and the study of *A Course in Miracles*. It is also a tangible reality thanks to the help of wonderful beings that supported me in the practical matters of editing and publishing this manuscript. My gratitude goes to my son Diego Ramos who designed the cover, helped edit and uploaded the book for publication.

I also want to acknowledge all of my clients who opened their hearts, minds, souls and shared their experiences with me. My appreciation to all of you, the readers, who made this book possible by your desire to connect to the greater Truth of your self-worth and identity.

Table of Contents

Introduction: Why Do We Define Self-Esteem?

We recognize that there is variability of meaning in the words that we use. We have and use dictionaries for this reason. We understand that our heritage, cultural background and experiences color our interpretations of the words we hear. And although we have been collectively conditioned by society in how we look at life, our individual perspective is nevertheless unique. This is because our experiences, the interpretations we give them and our response to them, are ours alone.

Our interpretations, the meaning we give to our experiences, shape our perspective. They powerfully direct how we see and value our current situation and our "self". In many ways, we can say that we are "a world onto ourselves". It is difficult for two people to see everything exactly the same, or agree on everything. It is as if we are looking out onto the same world while standing on top of different mountains.

From my mountain, full communication and understanding between people appears to be the exception and not the rule, since we can be looking at the same vista, but looking at it from different angles. Despite differences in our perspective, through this book I am humbly attempting to share with you a different point of view.

I attempt this because I have faith that deep connection and communication is completely possible, despite what my thinking says. I am aligning my faith with what I want to happen: the communication of a perspective that brings a permanent solution to the self-esteem problem.

My intention is to help you recognize your boundless true worth by looking at it from a spiritual angle. From this point of view, regard for you "self" is automatic and beyond question.

Perhaps you can see why this is a humble attempt. I will be using words and perception to help transcend these very things that shape our current view of our "self". This would not be possible without recognizing that there is something within all of us that resonates with the truth of our worth, despite appearances to the contrary.

May this book be a mirror that reflects back your true worth and may you receive this understanding with certainty.

Chapter 1: What is Self-Esteem?

First of all, let's understand that the word "self-esteem" represents an idea. When we speak it, we are trying to describe something we notice about how we are feeling about our "self" as a result of an evaluation. "Self-esteem" is an indicator of how much we are valuing our "self" and implies measurement. We often include the words "low" or "high" when referring to self-esteem because they measure the amount of "self" regard on a scale that measures worth and value.

The American Heritage Dictionary defines self-esteem simply as "pride in oneself". But, the dictionary's definition of "pride" is quite varied: self-respect; taking pleasure or satisfaction in one's work; achievements or possessions and conceit.

In addition to "pride" having many different meanings, it is fundamentally expressing a feeling. Our experience demonstrates that our emotions are not permanent. Emotions can be fickle and unstable. We can feel great about our "self", lose that feeling unexpectedly, and then have to look for ways to get it back. Perhaps over time a general negative undertone can settle in and then, we rarely seem to feel good about our "self".

It follows that in order to have and maintain stable, high self-esteem; we would need to keep feeling "proud" of our "self" continuously. This sets up a requirement to see our "self" in a positive light constantly. And while many books on self-esteem address what individuals can do to improve or build self-esteem to sustain one's positive regard, or make it stronger, the problem of consistency often remains.

How can we continuously keep seeing our "self" positively, so we can keep feeling good? From a spiritual perspective, there is a way to understand the "self" that can help us do this. We can learn to not just see our "self" in a positive light but ultimately *identify* with the positive light that is within us always, and truly reflects our self-worth.

If you are only looking to build your self-esteem, you are accepting that it has an unstable, changing nature. Besides the fact that building anything requires work, and more work to sustain it, what certainty do you have that what you build will not be torn down?

We say, "His self-esteem took a hit when he was passed up for the promotion." Or, "She lost her self-esteem when her partner left her." From this viewpoint, failing to get or keep what we want has the potential to crush our self-esteem and hurt us. Self-esteem is turned into a frail creature that needs protecting so we can be safe from emotional pain.

I want to suggest that if self-esteem is a problem for you, it is partly due to the existing definition that sees it as impermanent, frail and in need of building.

You may also notice that you might have high regard for your "self" in some areas of your life, but not in others. So it would be easy to conclude, "It's not possible to feel good about my "self" in all places and at all times." This brings up issues which I will address later in this book: why does our "esteem" change with our circumstances? And more importantly, how are we defining our "self" that makes this variability even possible?

In the next chapters we will also look at important ideas that need to be understood to be able to come to a greater appreciation of our true "Self". We will explore perception, what it is and how it works; how our mind evaluates to conclude what is worthy and valuable; "self" images we make of our "Self"; what is true and what is Truth; how we hijack our "Self" by holding false identifications and how the conclusions we make about our "self" seem to give or take away our worth.

Chapter 2: Perception and Our Memory Database

Have you, or someone you know, ever looked for something in the refrigerator or on a shelf and concluded, "It is not here." Then someone else comes to help, and there it is, right in front of your eyes! This is a familiar experience. I've had it many times and so have my children.

When this happens to me, I notice that my mind already has some idea or an image of what it is looking for. My eyes simply scan the area doing a matching game, looking for the object that fits the picture. Our mind holds information from past experiences and uses it as reference to help us identify things. When our mind is narrowly focused by past information and looks for an exact match, it can limit our ability to see things that may be different.

For example, if we hold a memory of the location, shape or color of the mayonnaise jar we used last time, we may fail to give proper attention to other locations and bypass slightly different looking jars. In this situation, our eyes are automatically scouting the area for an exact match to the memory. If the mayonnaise jar that is now in the refrigerator is another brand, a smaller size, or is in a different shelf, our eyes can easily miss it. We will conclude, "It is not here."

In this case, it may not even occur to us to look behind other jars that got put in front of it. The mayonnaise could be literally in front of our eyes, but we don't see it. It is like visiting friends we have not seen or been in contact with for years. It doesn't occur to us that their situation and address could have changed. We show up at their doorstep expecting them to be there, but they are not. They have moved. We trusted old information and could not find them where we looked.

Our perception is especially prone to get confused and miss things when we are under stress, rushing or in fear. There is a very good reason for this. Fear can activate our survival instincts. They are very primitive and focus our perception on finding the threat to our life. However, the threats in modern life have changed. For most of us, there is no hungry wolf lurking behind the bushes ready to attack, "I just can't find my cell phone!" Granted, to some of us this can feel like our survival is at stake, but we don't need to fight, run or play dead here.

What we need in this situation is to stay calm and think clearly to look for the phone. Being free of stress will also help our memory retrieve the information of where we put the phone last. It is precisely because our primitive instincts are looking for something that is not there, something that can hurt or kill us that they get in the way. We often miss the information that would help us find the phone because it is not a match to our primitive definition of threat. So the perceiving mind will dismiss pertinent information, both in trying to remember where we left it, and in noticing information in our environment associated to the location of the cell phone.

Let me illustrate with a personal experience:

One day engrossed in my job responsibilities, I lost track of time. I looked up at the clock and thought, "I'm going to be late for my next job!" Instinctively I stood up and quickly got ready to go. But I couldn't find my keys. I was positive I had put them in my top desk drawer. But they were not there!

Anxiety filled my chest as the clock ticked and I looked and looked! Finally giving up, I called my husband for a spare key. The next day, calm and rested, I opened my desk drawer and guess what I saw? My keys, exactly where I had left them!

We have all had similar experiences where we got caught up in the "threat" of the situation and couldn't see or think clearly. While this can be frustrating, it is part of the inherent glitches in our perception. It is important to understand how perception works because we will be applying this understanding later when we look at the negative views that we hold of our "self".

The biggest problem with our self-esteem and how we see our "self" is that our perception works from old and inaccurate self-assessments and evaluations, and tenaciously holds them as truth, often despite having evidence to the contrary.

All information coming in from our experiences and through our senses is stored in our subconscious mind. The mechanism for retrieving information from there, we call memory. We can imagine the information in our subconscious mind to be in a giant computer database. It stores everything we have learned, experienced and concluded to be true and false. As we grow, the information increases, getting updated or corrected and/or deleted, as new information comes in. This is what learning is. As the words, pictures, feelings, experiences, beliefs, sounds, tastes etc. in our database change, so does our perspective and how we see our "self" and the world.

Our database holds not just individually learned information but also group and ancestral memories, beliefs, experiences, etc. Yet, every individual's database has its own unique flavor to it. No two individuals have made sense of their life exactly in the same way. This makes our perception very personal.

That we can relate to each other's experiences means that there is a significant amount of common information in our databases. Many of our experiences and the learning and conclusions from them have been similar. There is wide agreement in our individual perceptions, though not complete. It follows that our perceptions will have much more in common with those of our own group, generation and culture, and their teachings will be included as part of the personal way we see things.

For example, the standards for physical beauty and attractiveness vary between cultures. Some African cultures perceive a thin woman to be unattractive. Also, in past centuries people perceived the world as flat. This way of looking at the earth was passed down generation to generation. When children looked out to sea and saw the flat horizon their eyes confirmed a culturally accepted but inaccurate perspective!

Now we can easily see the perceptual error people were making in believing the world was flat, but when individuals first began to point out that the earth was round; they were judged by many to be crazy. It took time for this new perspective to gain acceptance and replace what had been accepted as true before.

What I hope you recognize is that how we see things, and what we see, is very much influenced by our past learning and how up to date the database information in our perceiving mind is. This applies to how we see our "self" too. It is very possible that we are holding old and inaccurate information that is skewing our "self" perception in a negative direction.

Chapter 3: Perception and Distortion

There is one more very important point to note in how our perception makes errors. You may find it a little unsettling, but it needs addressing because it can cause deep distortion in how we see our "self".

Take a look at this example:

My husband and I were watching _Toy Story III_. Towards the end of the movie something did not make sense to me because I could clearly recall that the young man put his cowboy toy named Woody, in the box that was labeled "attic". I mentioned this to my husband and he said, "No, he put it in the box labeled 'college'."

Because I could run that part of the movie in my mind and see Woody going into the "attic" box, I believed I was right. I was so sure that what I saw in my mind was correct that I insisted we rewind the movie. So, we watched that part again.

Wow! I found it really difficult to believe what my eyes were showing me! Woody did go into the box for "college." I was dumbfounded. How could I have been so sure and been completely wrong?

For me, it was curious to observe that I chose to believe what I *thought* and could see *in my mind*: Woody going into the "attic" box, and would not believe my eyes when they were seeing the truth: Woody going into the "college" box! I seemed silly how I placed more faith in what my perceiving mind was showing me, rather than in the information coming from my physical senses and my husband. But, my husband was not so amused and with good reason, I might add.

To understand what happened in my *Toy Story III* example, let's explore further our informational database and what happens when new information is coming in. Like I said before, as we grow and learn we correct and let go of some of the information in our database. We stop believing in Santa Claus and the Tooth Fairy for example. Information is revised, updated and released. Information that survives this continual process of revision and updating gets reinforced with time and experience.

21

The long-standing, stronger beliefs left intact in the process of learning become foundational cornerstones to our identity and world perspective. They provide perceptual stability to our "self" and our life, even if they are incorrect, much like the belief that the world was flat that endured for centuries. While we can still shift our perspective and revise our foundational beliefs, it becomes harder because they have been getting reinforced over and over in time becoming more deeply imprinted into our perception.

Perceptual stability is assured through a subconscious filtering mechanism made up of our foundational beliefs. Most all new information must pass through these perceptual filters. Information from new experiences will get evaluated by our foundational beliefs before it is accepted into our database for storage. If the new information matches the existing foundational beliefs, it is allowed in. But if it does not, it may be ignored, dismissed or distorted to force a match.

Distortion will happen if the new information puts into question and challenges an existing, subconscious foundational belief that we have taken on as part of our identity. This is called identification and I will describe it in detail in another chapter. Keeping the foundational belief from being revised becomes a priority for our perceiving mind because it is seen as a part of us. Whatever threatens to do away with the belief is felt to be a personal threat to who we are. In these situations, fabricating a revised version of reality becomes justified and necessary in our mind, as in the case of my *Toy Story III* example.

It is important to recognize the power the perceiving mind has to distort truth when it imagines and presents a different picture of reality to us, and we believe it. When we subconsciously choose to believe our imagination over the facts, we lose touch with reality. This blinds us to the whole truth of what is present before us.

It is quite astonishing to witness the length our perceiving mind is willing to go to hold on to some of its cherished beliefs. It is like going to look for the mayonnaise jar in the refrigerator and because it is not where we believe it should be, we pick up the jar of pickles that is in its place and imagining it to be the mayonnaise. We do this in order to keep our belief intact and not see that our thinking is incorrect.

Clearly the pickles are still the pickles, but in our mind we can *make believe* they are the mayonnaise.

Accepting new facts that revise or invalidate what we believe to be true is the basis for learning and the mechanism that updates the content of our database. When this takes place, our perception is also revised and we see things differently. If this does not happen, we miss an opportunity for possible growth.

A strong pattern of resistance to updating our foundational beliefs keeps our perceptions stable but distorted; maintaining how we want to keep seeing situations can keep us from seeing reality as it is. To maintain this distortion requires mental energy and can take a toll on our mental faculties over time. I have seen this with my mother who is in the late stages of Alzheimer's.

A very quick example of what I witnessed is the time my mother was giving casual advice to my sister. She said to her, "If your husband raises his voice at you, just make believe you didn't hear him." This was her strategy, and one she believed would serve her daughter well, for coping with some of the unpleasant situations she perhaps felt powerless to change.

I realize that there may be resistance to some of these ideas for some of you. This reaction is not out of line with the point I am making: when some of our foundational beliefs are being challenged, it can feel uncomfortable and even scary. It is precisely this disturbance that we need to notice when new information is presented to us. It can be a signal of resistance that is telling us that one or more of our foundational beliefs are being challenged.

It can be difficult to keep our perceiving mind always open to change. It may feel like we are waiting for an earthquake to happen and that our stable house of perception anchored by our foundational beliefs, could come crumbling down. And yet it is very important to understand how distortion happens so we can catch our perceiving mind doing it. In my experience, distortion and identification with our beliefs is at the root of our self-esteem problems: believing a negative distorted version of the truth with regard to our true value and identity. But here too is a permanent solution offered, as I will point out later.

To reiterate, our foundational beliefs get protected to keep our world view stable from the instability that is felt when we go through big changes that shock our belief system. We experience loss, break-ups and catastrophe and these experiences intensify our fear of change. Very few people welcome drastic change for this reason. It forces revision on our foundational beliefs and our identity gets shaken to its core.

Distortion helps us to maintain an illusion of stability, control and helps us to feel safer in a world that appears to be threatening and constantly changing. Many times, we choose a sense of safety from our fears at the expense of reality and of us not being able to see the whole truth.

The resistance to believing my eyes when they saw Woody going into the "college" box was coming from my existing beliefs doing their best to avoid deletion. Their voices objecting, "That can't be right! A college student would not, and should not, be taking his childhood toy with him to college! It most definitely belongs in the 'attic' box!!"

These beliefs literally rewrote the story. They were looking to my eyesight to find a match of support, not for contradiction! Although this process took place out of my conscious awareness, looking back on it helped me uncover the subconscious beliefs and see how much influence my perceiving mind has on what I see, and don't see, in my experiences.

Perhaps this is still sounding strange and your beliefs are also objecting. That is fine. Notice how easy it is to get attached to our way of seeing things and to how we want things to be. This also supports a feeling of stability and safety in our perceptual world.

My example with *Toy Story III* shows how loyal we can be to some of our beliefs and internal pictures. Once our perceiving mind concludes something is fundamentally true, and holds vivid memories of happenings that support that conclusion, it can take a lot to change our mind. In addition, many of our foundational beliefs hide deep in the subconscious part of our mind, further assuring their survival. However, to bring change to our "self" perception, we need to bring into consciousness those beliefs responsible for our negative thinking and reactions, so we can consciously change them.

When you are having issues with self-esteem, you are seeing your "self" from a negative perspective. What is your perception finding or fabricating in your mind? Are you holding beliefs that say: "I am unwanted; I am stupid; there is something wrong with me; I can't do anything right; I am worthless; I am a looser; I am unlovable; I am invisible; I am a burden; I am broken; I am bad; I am a sinner; I am unheard; I get blamed for everything; I'm undeserving of good things; etc.?"

Conscious and deliberate intervention is needed with these types of beliefs that form our negative self-image. Otherwise, they will keep strengthening themselves through the perceiving mind's filtering process.

I worked with a client grieving the death of his spouse. He had taken out a box of old letters that his wife had written to him over the years. He noticed that many of the loving things she had written him, he had forgotten. He wondered why it had been so easy to remember her negative comments, but not the positive ones that he re-read in her letters.

When we hold negative self-images of our "self", our perceiving mind will be trying to find a match when we look in the refrigerator, called our life. My client remembered the negative comments because that was what matched his database beliefs about himself, at that time. Now that he saw himself in a better light, he was able to notice his past perceptual bias towards her negative comments.

We find what we seek and our foundational beliefs play a powerful part in the seeking. Here we can recognize that since our perceptions are focused on finding a match to what they represent, we can consciously intervene when we are finding negativity. By choosing to consciously maintain a positive perspective in new situations, and opening our mind to new information that can revise and delete negative foundational beliefs, we can help correct our perception.

Correcting our negative beliefs is like clearing away the fog that hides the bright sunshine. Now the light is able to shine through and we can see the matching good things in our life. Once we clear enough of the foundational negative beliefs, a positive view point will begin to emerge and reinforce itself.

Chapter 4: Blocks to Correcting Our Perception

To correct our perception, or clear misperception, we need to observe our thinking so we can find the negative underlying beliefs and question their validity so they can be updated or let go. This process can feel threatening for various reasons. I already mentioned that perception works very hard to maintain the appearance of stability. Any practice that looks to question the truth of what is in our database to correct it, can often feel like an attack, if we perceive correction as a negative judgment on us. Again, any type of fear or resistance around this process only serves to protect the existing negative beliefs that need changing.

If we feel unhappy and have problems with self-esteem, change is clearly needed to how we are seeing our "self". To get to the bottom of our self-esteem issues, we need to look at the negative self-images that we believe our "self" is, and which are stored in our subconscious database. These self-images got labeled as true, then accepted into our database and now get used as reference for interpreting new situations in our life.

With an understanding of how perception works, we can revisit the assumptions we made when we accepted those beliefs as true to, then change our mind, and see our "self" differently. This is how we bring about change in our world perception, by changing the information in the database within.

I have been examining the content of my database information since college. Also, for the past seven years I have worked with clients uncovering and revising the content of their databases. What often shows up on this path of clearing misperception is emotional pain. When we explore our negative views, we inevitably find buried hurt. Not too many people welcome these discoveries. Yet they are the key to shifting our perception.

We need to understand that emotional pain got buried, often at a very young age, precisely because we were not able to process it and release it. Emotional pain says nothing negative or personal about us. If we approach the exploration of our databases like an archeological excavation to find buried dinosaur bones that are of no danger or consequence to us now, the easier and more exciting our discoveries will be.

Keep in mind that any layers of emotion surrounding our deep hurts needs to be released for healing to take place. These emotions are the glue anchoring the negative "self" beliefs in our database. For this reason, techniques like EFT (Emotional Freedom Techniques) target them for healing. I will introduce EFT in the last chapter, let me just say that releasing negative emotions can be done much quicker and easier than previously believed.

Burying hurt is a strategy that many of us have used to make our "self" feel better. Unfortunately, it has its drawbacks. Burying the hurt doesn't release it. It can fester inside disturbing our wellbeing. For some of us, our buried, emotional dinosaur bones have turned into petroleum oil, slippery and hard to contain. The negativity spews out when we least expect it.

You may have heard someone say, "He pushed my buttons and I exploded." Something in their situation triggered off an uncontrolled reaction. It can feel like a remote detonator got pushed and our *defenses* came down, allowing our imprisoned emotions to burst through like angry animals out of control.

Many times we feel just as scared as those witnessing our overreactions because we have no idea where and who is pushing these "buttons" and how to stop them from getting pushed again. We can see that these reactions are not in line with what the situation called for. But, we are often left feeling powerless to change them.

The triggers that bring up old hurt can be anything: a sensory cue, what someone said, how they said it, the tone of their voice, the way they looked at us, the expression on their face, the particular place, a color, a sound and even someone's smile. Sometimes a small trigger can be what we refer to as, "The last straw that broke the camel's back."

The triggers are unconscious red flags that wave to us because they are supposed to get our attention, emotions are not meant to be buried or locked up. Emotions are expressions. Expressions need to have their say and want to be heard. It is not so much that others need to acknowledge them, sometimes this is necessary, but their message is primarily for us. This is how we can learn to not be afraid of feeling our emotions; help heal our past hurts; be more accepting of our whole "self" and come to live in peace with our past.

Emotional overreactions are a sign that past events and the associated hurt have not completely healed. The hurt is still raw. Until we have peace around our hurtful past, it will exert power over our present experiences and project fear into our future. Our perception will be keenly focused on what, in the present situation, is similar to the past hurtful experiences, believing that by "watching out" for these cues, we can protect our "self" from more pain. Unfortunately, focusing our attention on what we want to avoid means our attention will find that: what it is seeking to avoid, and so we often find what we consciously don't want.

This is similar to the idea of the *Law of Attraction* which says, "Like attracts like." The reason for this has to do with how our past events get associated to feelings in our memory. Our memory uses emotions to connect experiences that have a like feel. The feelings are triggered by the sensory information in the new experience and because we are not aware of these triggers, it feels like the emotions come up automatically.

When we encounter the sensory trigger in a new situation, our memory also pulls up the matching past event that has a similar feel. The perceiving mind will then focus on specific information from the new experience that makes a match to the past unresolved one. Therefore, we perceive the new situation to be similar to the old and so we say, "Like attracts like" experiences.

However, when a new event *reminds* us of a past event, it is not necessarily because the two events are really alike, but because there is matching triggering information in the new situation. Our perception brings up the past feelings and makes the new situation appear and feel similar. Remember the fear around not finding the cell phone? It is not because the situation of losing the cell phone was really about survival, but in our mind it reminded us and brought up the feelings of a past survival experience.

Our emotional reactions are often automatic conditioned responses based on our past experiences and existing beliefs, and not necessarily to the reality of life. If I believe, "I can't live without my cell phone", the loss of it will trigger a survival reaction. In my mind, I have made the phone a necessity to life, not because it will really kill me not to have it, but because I have made it seem this way and believed it.

The idea of survival and the fear of death that is a part of it are part of some of the deepest and oldest programs stored in our database. The fight, flight or freeze reactions have been getting reinforced since the time of primitive man and before. These responses are so ingrained, long-standing and habitual that they are literally automatic, and so they have become instincts.

I sit quietly typing on my computer. Unexpectedly, I hear a sudden noise. I tense up with an automatic, fearful and contracted sensation down the middle of my body. A glass slipped from the stack of dishes in the kitchen sink. I relax, releasing my breath and I return to the obvious safety and comfort of my modern kitchen.

Why do I still hold such fearful reactions? I have never experienced any physical survival threats to my life. To me, it would make more sense that after living securely and comfortably for fifty years, my survival fears would have dissipated and left me. But wait, I grew up witnessing countless acts of violence and destruction since I was a child watching television and movies.

Isn't it interesting that my database had little problem accepting such violent information? Why isn't it pulling its "distorting" and "not finding a match" tricks here? Could it be that it is matching and reinforcing beliefs that have been subconsciously getting supported for thousands of years that say, "I live in a violent and dangerous world?

Much of our modern entertainment provides the opportunity to find plenty of survival matches, and I have vicariously reinforced them, often on a daily basis. After all, I have been not just willing to subject my "self" to witnessing screen violence, but I have valued it enough to pay for it.

Take a look at the type of entertainment you engage in. What beliefs are getting matched and reinforced by what you witness? Are these beliefs you truly want to externally reinforce?

I can't emphasize enough how deeply implanted our survival fears and beliefs are. They have stayed with us and flourished, despite our industrial growth, rise in standard of living and technological advancement. In general, can we feel any safer today than people living in the 1700's? Does having met basic food, clothing and shelter needs and piling leisure and comfort on top, really keep us from experiencing survival fears?

My mother experienced severe poverty growing up. Her whole village went through a famine brought on by an outbreak of Mad Cow disease in the 1940's in Mexico. But her economic situation drastically improved when we moved to California in 1968. For many years, she was able to experience abundance in all areas of her life, including having full ownership of a four bedroom home.

Yet, the external changes to her social economic reality were not enough to revise and clear her existing childhood foundational beliefs around scarcity and survival. The behavior patterns supported by these beliefs continued to be displayed through her Alzheimer's. She feared that toilet paper, or anything else, would be stolen if left out in plain sight. She would hide everything to keep it safe. So when she went to look for those things, she didn't remember she had hidden them, and concluded that they had been stolen. In many ways, our beliefs are more powerful in defining and influencing our experiences than the physical reality we live in.

This is unfortunate when it comes to our deeply imprinted survival beliefs. They continue to powerfully filter our modern life experiences of ease and convenience needing to find something threatening to overcome. Our perceiving mind can make almost anything look like a threat to us.

We can take words, gestures, remarks and the look someone gives us to be dangerous daggers. Exams, bills, dating, our children's demands, criticism, judgment, disagreements, etc. become threats or attacks that need to be survived.

In fact, words or actions that discredit our respectability, honor or reputation can feel like personal attacks to our "self" and self-esteem. Whoever said, "Sticks and stones can break my bones, but words can never hurt me.", was talking about the physical world and not perception. We no longer need spears and rocks to hurt each other, we throw some choice words or hand gestures packed with negative meaning to do emotional damage.

Present experiences continue to feed fears and provide proof of our vulnerability to attack, confirming a self-image that says "I am weak and vulnerable to hurt." Can a powerless view of our "self" that supports a belief that says, "I am a victim living in a dangerous and violent world" accept the immense power that can comes with recognizing that changing our perception has the effect of changing our life?

In the next chapter I will explain the role of personal interpretation in perception and give more examples of how misperceptions are formed. I want to help you understand how negative and fearful perceptions of our "self" are just conditioned, ingrained and pain fueled points of view, and not Truth from a spiritual perspective.

It is necessary to be able to let go of any fear or resistance to looking at our negative self-perceptions. They are hidden from our sight in the subconscious part of our mind for a good reason: we want to believe that what we can't see is not there. In this way, we can't change what we don't want to see. Yet their powerful effects will continue to be felt and reflected in the quality of our experiences.

It is harder to deny our negative self-perceptions at the level of experience where their effects are felt, though it is still possible through distortion. And though distortion is an option, it is very hard to keep fooling ourselves forever.

Chapter 5: Interpretation and Reaction

I used to work doing Spanish-English translating and interpreting for schools and businesses. I would read or listen to the meaning of the words of one language, holding it in mind, while finding the words that best expressed that meaning in the other language. But you can see that an unskilled or biased interpreter, one that doesn't know both languages well and cannot stay objective, can easily distort the communication. It is often said, "Something got lost in the translation."

When we are trying to communicate with someone and we are unable to come to an understanding, it can feel like we are speaking different languages. This type of problem is also a perception problem. Our subconscious database of information sits like a hired interpreter between them and us. It picks up the information coming in, runs it through its filters, and gives us the interpreted version of what was said.

Our interpreter is always with us giving us its interpretation of what is happening in all areas of our life. Our conscious mind uses the interpreted information to make decisions, taking the information in good faith and assuming that it is accurate. But more often than we care to see, we are misled and act on misinterpretations due to the limitations and biases of our database filters.

Realizing that our perception is not always objective or skilled in interpreting certain situations accurately, will help us to be more compassionate with the mess that results from the misunderstandings. We may look back at our trespasses wondering, "What in the world was I thinking, to say/do such terrible things?" That is precisely what we want to investigate, our thinking and database interpretations of the situation.

It is easy to look back on a problem event and judge our "self" harshly over what took place. But we need to understand how our database was interpreting the situation to see that we were acting in good faith believing our database interpretations to be true. We want to notice what meaning our interpretations gave us that triggered the feelings and the actions/words we now regret.

Look at a past event where you said or did something you would not do again. How was your perceiving mind interpreting the situation? What beliefs and fears are driving this interpretation? Can you see that your actions took direction from these thoughts and feelings?

Given how you perceived the situation in the moment it happened, could you see another option for your behavior? Most of the time, we see no other option. But if you did, what interpretations kept you from acting on the other options? Much of what we regret occurs because our interpreter is speaking fear to us through the point of view of a young, inexperienced or scared and hurt child and this perspective takes us over.

Don't underestimate the power of your interpretations. Your behavior takes direction from what your database interprets as true in the moment. Our over-reactions are not without explanation or out of control. They only appear that way because the interpreting happens mostly at the subconscious level. There are tools and practices available to us now for making what is unconscious, conscious. We can learn to pay attention to our feelings and reactions to trace what is giving rise to them and find the subconscious associations and interpretations that will need correcting.

Let me give you some simple examples of the power of interpretation:

Once in a while when I cook, my youngest daughter walks into the kitchen. The smells catch her off guard, she reacts showing disgust on her face, and unable to speak, quickly leaves. While these smells are offensive to her, they are enticing to me. They remind me of good tasting food. They bring up fond images of eating and enjoying time spent with family around the dinner table. It is these pleasant associations that give those smells a positive interpretation for me. They represent something very different to me than to my daughter. We can wonder, "Is any smell really pleasant or unpleasant on its own?"

Once I attended a Halloween party where they put out closed boxes labeled "eyeballs", "intestines", etc. I put my hand through a hole in the box labeled "eyeballs". It felt so gross! The information from my sense of touch matched what I imagined eyeballs could feel like. I was convinced this was an accurate interpretation and reacted accordingly. After all, I could not think of anything else that could feel round, slimy and wet. Without previous experience touching eyeballs, and without information from my sight and taste, the "eyeball" label was a good interpretation. It was believable and I was tricked, but in reality I was touching round, peeled grapes.

There is an element of fun in innocently fooling others and getting fooled. Maybe it reminds us of being kids. My brother tricked his kids into eating pinto beans. When they looked at the beans initially, they refused to eat them. He mashed them up and told them that it was "Meat beaten to a pulp." They believed his interpretation and ate the beans just fine!

Chapter 6: Foundational Impressions

As we saw with the pinto bean example, kids can be fooled quite easily and accept what to us are obvious distortions of the truth. This happens because their database contains few foundational beliefs to sort out new information. On the positive side, because of this they learn quickly, remain curious and keep an open mind. They can't filter out fantastic beliefs like Santa Claus, the Tooth Fairy, the Easter Bunny, etc., since just about everything is possible, new, amazing and outrageous to them.

For these reasons, many of our early childhood experiences form the roots of our later deeply seated foundational beliefs. Conclusions we reach as children, regardless of their accuracy or plausibility, can imprint deeply into our very impressionable young database. The resulting beliefs then become pivotal in how we come to regard and think of our "self". It also happens that we can inherit foundational beliefs or views of our "self" and reinforce these in time.

Think of a young child's first encounter with a dog. This experience will be foundational because it will serve as a reference for the next encounter. If the initial experience is painful, perhaps because the dog bit the child, this memory will be infused with fear. Our primitive brain will govern that memory, since it's in command of our survival. Traumatic moments like this become the domain of this part of our mind. The primitive mind takes over the more rational thinking part in these situations and later gets re-triggered by similar situations if the trauma has not healed.

Depending on the child's interpretations, only certain types of dogs or all dogs in general, could be incriminated and labeled as dangerous. Expecting pain to come from dogs, the child will instinctively react by moving away, attempting to avoid an encounter with another one.

While another experience with a different dog offers the possibility of a different and better result, if the child has not released the initial fear, there will be resistance to this new opportunity.

Even if the child's next dog experience is not avoided, as long as the initial fear remains from the earlier experience, the odds of a repeat trauma go up. The dog will sense the child's fear, increasing the chance that it will bark and react as if the child is an intruder.

Again, "like" will attract "like". When this happens, the existing association of dog and pain will be further reinforced in the child's mind. For this reason childhood negative experiences lay the foundation for our adult belief system and perspective. The conclusions and interpretations reached by the child through these experiences will impact the rest of their life if not revised or cleared at some point. They lay the ground for possibly attracting future similar experiences.

Imagine you are a toddler and you hear your mother screaming loudly. You feel her fear as you see her terrified expression and notice what her wide open eyes are starring at, a black little thing called a spider. She is communicating to you, "Danger, danger! There is the threat!" Your small primitive mind easily accepts her convincing interpretation and concludes that, it must be true, spiders are dangerous!

On the other hand, maybe you had already played happily in the garden with a few spiders and their webs. Or maybe Dad came to help Mom, got a tissue, and calmly picked up the spider and put it outside. This additional information is pointing out that perhaps spiders are not dangerous. This other information may be enough to release the fear that came up from hearing your mother scream, or not.

To let go of the fear of spiders completely, a toddler will still need to make some sense of Mom's terror. They will need to find an interpretation that explains her fearful reaction. Remember, a toddler is going to heavily weigh all information coming from Mom and Dad because they are dependent on them. The toddler cannot simply disregard Mom's fearful reaction. It is possible that the toddler will conclude something about Mom, or begin to form a general conclusion about women and men such as: "Mom is not very strong, little things scare her"; "Men don't get scared, but women do" or "Dad is stronger than Mom."

Are such conclusions fine for a toddler? Yes, they make a scary and confusing world more predictable and help them to feel safe. Could these conclusions be unhelpful later in their adult life? Yes! Depending on which conclusions got reinforced in their later years, the now adult could be afraid of spiders; see themselves as weak when they scream or feel scared; or devalue their "self" by making the judgment that they are acting "like a girl" when they feel fear. All these would contribute to a negative "self" evaluation, and more so, for a man's self-esteem due to accepted cultural expectations and beliefs between genders.

Chapter 7: How Distorted Perceptions Gain Acceptance

In general, foundational views not revised or released become stronger as we age since they serve as filters for keeping out non-conforming information. Unless we make an effort to stay curious and keep an open mind, our foundational beliefs can keep us expecting and experiencing our future similarly to our past. Our perceiving mind would then shield us from opening our mind to new possibilities for our future. This would solidify our existing perspective even more, making the future just an extension of the past. For some of us, future predictability and stability gives us a feeling of safety and is therefore desirable. However, it also keeps us stuck and resistant to the deep change we desperately need and want in our life.

If you have difficulty with self-esteem, you will need to examine and question your foundational beliefs in order to bring about change. In particular, the negative beliefs about your "self" will need examining. Some of the most powerful beliefs, both positive and negative, start with "I am": I am ugly, I am intelligent, I am a looser, I am successful, I am the clothes I wear, I am a college graduate, I am a woman, I am a minority, I am a high school drop-out, I am a mother, I am a cancer survivor, etc. Be ready to look at them fearlessly. Notice the effects they've had, and continue to have on your life. The fear of examining them only keeps them in place. Don't be surprised if some of the negative "I am" beliefs are protected and held in place by past emotional pain, fears, and an unwillingness to forgive. This is how they have endured and made themselves at home in your mind.

Take this example on how difficult it can be to want to change our beliefs:

I had a very nice high school teacher who adored me, perhaps because I fit the model of the ideal student, eager to learn and please. But there was something this teacher could not reconcile in her mind. I was Mexican.

She would ask me, "Are you sure you are Mexican?"

A bit uncomfortably I would reply, "Yes."

I could feel this was not the right answer she wanted to hear. But, I could not say "No." There was no question as to where I was born.

Nevertheless she would insist, "No, you can't be Mexican, you must be Spanish!"

I sensed her mind's conflict. She really liked me, but there was something about me that did not fit in with her definition of "Mexican". So, rather than question and perhaps revise her definition, she decided to change me, in her mind at least.

The perceiving part of our mind does not care if we deceive ourselves, as you also saw with the *Toy Story III* example. It can sometimes work very hard to protect whatever it has interpreted and defined as true. When faced with contradictory new information that would lead this part of our mind to question its existing definitions and views, it can easily choose to turn a blind eye to facts. However, our then reality gets distorted and we can turn our "self", others and the world into something it is not.

But remember distortion only happens in our mind, not in Truth. Could my teacher change me from being Mexican to Spanish? No, she could only do that in her mind, not in reality. Could I really change the *Toy Story III* movie? No, I could imagine Woody going into the "attic" box, and I could believe that what I saw in my imagination was true, but I did not change the movie or the fact that Woody went into the "college" box.

Distortion cannot change reality in Truth. However, it does disturb the ease and peacefulness of our relationships and the quality of our life. Those around us witnessing the distortion are usually confused by our reactions and often not amused. In fact, if they don't understand the glitches in perception, they could easily react with annoyance, frustration or anger when we are having difficulty seeing the truth and may misinterpret the situation or take it personal.

The ability of our mind to make something up and then believe it to be truth is referred to as "illusion" or "Maya", in the Buddhist tradition. Maya forms a distorted version or story of reality that we accept as true. It is a skewed representation of what *is* because our past definitions and interpretations are the standards for filtering and deciding what is true in the present situation.

It is like drinking water from an outside well that pumps water into our kitchen. The well water is perfectly pure but the water pipes have been gradually corroding over time and allowing impurities to get in. Fortunately, the water faucet in the kitchen has a filter, but unfortunately, it has never been cleaned because no one is aware such a filter exists.

Generations come and go. They drink the faucet water thinking it is clean. They have no memory of the taste of the pure well water, so they keep drinking what comes out believing that it is free of impurities.

No one that tastes the pure well water is fooled into believing that the water coming out from the faucet is pure. But without this reference, or the awareness that there is a filter that needs to be cleaned on a regular basis, the house inhabitants keep drinking the contaminated water believing it is pure. In this manner, the taste of pure water is gradually distorted and its original taste, or truth, is lost.

But again it is not really lost, only hidden by the dirty filter. The fresh well water is still pure and getting pumped to the house. The filter needs cleaning or the inhabitants can go directly to the well. Once the filter is cleaned, the quality of the water coming out of the faucet will match very closely, the purity of the water from its source.

We can see that there has never been a problem with the well water; the problem has been the lack of awareness of the corroding pipes (perceptual distortion) and the filter that needs periodic cleaning (database information that needs revising and deleting).

In a similar way, small negative distortions have been introduced to our "self" perception over time and have gone unnoticed. Bias has been gradually accepted as real and true. This has happened mostly out of our conscious awareness through misinterpretations handed down by our clan, culture and religious teachings. We have accepted these misinterpretations as truth, not understanding the distortion process and the inaccuracies that have accumulated in our database.

Take a look at the interpretations you are giving to your behaviors, reactions and your "self"? The interpretations are like the faucet water. What kind of taste does it leave in your mouth? Is it really fresh and pure? If not, perhaps it is time to look at your perception filter and clean it up?

Chapter 8: Identification and Questioning Our Thinking

We have been trained to value and follow the part of our mind that thinks, analyzes, plans and forms perspectives. In fact, many of our parents warned and insisted that we must always think before we act. This was supposed to be for our own good and safety. However, for decision-making and in particular for making major life decisions, we need to take advice not just from the thinking part of our mind. Often, the desires of our heart and soul can be more important. Otherwise, these decisions and the life that results will lack the deep fulfillment that so many of us crave.

We spend many years in school developing our thinking intellect or focusing on gaining worldly smarts in order to solve our problems and help get us what we think we want. We have come to believe that having a keen intellect will ensure our safety, success and happiness in life.

We illicit and accept advice from experts and authority figures because we want to believe they always know best. We rely on our database intelligence and that of others' to help us survive the difficulties that face us. When this strategy fails us, we feel devastated and loose trust and confidence in our "self", others and life. But what has really failed us? It is an overreliance on our own ingenuity and the faith we put in the accumulation of data as the ultimate source of salvation from all of our problems.

Though we can give credit to our intelligence for many technological advances and for easing the need for hard physical labor, it has not been able to solve our longstanding problems of poverty, disease, war and unhappiness. Nevertheless, we have made this part of our perceiving mind very important to us and for good reason. Intelligence, which includes our database system of information, holds the maps and rules for living life as prescribed by those before us and their collective advice.

Unfortunately, we have placed so much trust on this intelligence that for the most part, we give it unrestricted freedom to run our life. Taking and following direction from our mind's stored rules and conventions is an unconscious habit for most of us. We have done this for so long, that it has become an automatic pilot, deciding which roads we travel in life without our full awareness.

Even if we have doubts about trusting our accumulated learning fully; perhaps because serious errors have been made in the past, it can appear as if it is all we have.

Let me give you an every-day example of how automatically listening to our thinking can steer us wrong and how inner guidance helps us:

On a brisk February morning I needed to make a trip to a bank in a nearby city. When I located the address on an internet map, the area looked familiar. Having traveled to this city a few times before and *thinking* I knew where the street Golf Course Drive was, I left feeling confident I would easily find my way.

As I drove on the highway I had a *picture* in my mind of which exit I needed to take. As I got closer to that exit, I noticed a different exit named "Willow and Golf Course Drive".

This was new information to me, and I didn't have time to revise my previous conclusion about which exit I was *supposed* to take. So, I got off at the next one as planned. I *figured* that even if this was not Golf Course Drive, it would intersect at the next cross street.

This was a comforting *thought,* but I soon realized it was wrong. The intersection ahead was not Golf Course Drive. So, I turned around and headed back to the previous exit on a side road, again being assured by my *thinking:* "Now, I'm pretty sure I know which street is going to be Golf Course Drive."

I drove up to an intersection just before the street that I was *now thinking* would be Golf Course Drive and stopped for a red light. I looked around for the name of the cross street but could not see it anywhere. As I did this, I caught myself talking out loud, "I have a *feeling* that this is the street I want." Without a second thought, I quickly switched lanes and turned. Within a couple of blocks I saw a long golf course! I laughed with relief. It made sense that a street named Golf Course Drive would have a golf course on it, and I was finally on the correct street!

So then I started looking for the building numbers, but couldn't find any. I saw a shopping center ahead but without any numbers to orient myself with.

I almost passed the shopping center, but I heard my *intuition* again and turned in. My perceiving mind was uncomfortable with my unexpected turn and justified it as "Ok" by *figuring* it would be easier to find the number for the shopping center or ask for directions. But none of that was necessary; to my left was a big ATM sign! The bank was there.

This experience showed me how readily I follow my thinking mind. It felt automatic. I was amazed at how it didn't occur to me to question how my thinking "knew" where to take me, if it wasn't *certain* it really knew. It only *thought* it knew. That is not certainty.

I believed my thinking mind was "pretty sure" it could find this bank without a problem, but how could it know for sure without having been there before? Even if I had seen the bank or been there before, I could have remembered incorrectly. Remember how wrong my thinking mind was with my *Toy Story III* example?

Again, I am not trying to say that we can't trust our thinking at all, I am grateful to use it in this moment to organize the ideas I want to communicate to you in this book. What I am questioning and what I want you to question is, "How important have I made my thinking and perception in my life?" And now that we see that there are glitches, "Am I comfortable and willing to have it automatically direct so many of my decisions?"

I saw that I had incorrectly believed I could find certainty in my thinking mind. But certainty is not found in perception and thinking, only beyond our beliefs. To know certainty we need to bypass the faucet filter and go drink of the well water that is the source of fresh and pure water. At the very least, if we clean our database filter our thinking will be more clear and accurate.

Here is another quick example of* thinking *I knew something but not with certainty:

On school days I make a sandwich for my son's lunch in the morning. Often, I make an extra one for my husband. One morning my husband said, "I'm leaving for work. Oh, I need to make a sandwich." I automatically replied, "I made you one."

We looked around the kitchen counters for the sandwich, it was not there. I had to re-evaluate my statement. Did I really make him one? I did not know with certainty that I had. I told him, "I *thought* I made one for you. I *want to believe* that I made one for you, but I don't know with certainty that I did." We both had a good laugh.

In my previous bank example, it would have been better for me to admit up front that I did not know with certainty where this bank was. My mind was led astray by *thinking* and *believing* that I did know. Can you remember a time that you were lead astray *thinking* or *believing* you knew something but not with certainty?

Recognizing I did not really know where I was going would have left my mind open to taking direction from the exit sign that said, "Willow and *Golf Course Drive*"!

I'm glad for that experience and the learning I received. The experience is also giving me a way to explain a very important idea, *identification*. It is the source of much of our suffering but fundamentally a misperception

In my search for the bank, I became identified with the thinking part of my mind; my "self" identity merged with it. It felt like there was no difference between *my thinking* and my "self". I couldn't question *my thinking* because I was *my thinking*. Reread the following part of a previous paragraph:

Recognizing I did not really know where I was going would have left my mind open to taking direction from the exit sign that said, "Willow and Golf Course Drive"!

Take note of when I used the word "I", then go back and replace the "I" with the words "my thinking".

Observe how seamlessly "I" assumed the identity of "my thinking". We unconsciously make "I" interchangeable with whatever we are identified with in the moment. That is identification.

Let me give you another example of identification:

Imagine that you won your state sweepstake consisting of your dream car! You are handed the key. It is gorgeous! You can see your smiling face reflected on its shiny surface as you run you hand over the hood and feel how smooth it is. Not a dent or speck of dust on it.

Eagerly, you open the door and get in. The smell of "new" permeates your nose. You get acquainted with the car's interior, turn on the engine and off you go feeling ten feet tall!

Deciding to stop at a store, you pull into a parking space. As you are about to open your car door, the woman in the next car on the passenger side is also opening her door. She opens her car door too wide and you hear and feel the vibrations made by impact, door hitting door.

What physical and/or emotional reaction are you feeling in this moment? Notice what part of your body is feeling this "impact". Did it feel like you were the one getting hit? Does it feel like what happened to your car is personal?

If you felt the imaginary "impact", your consciousness was merged with your dream car. Or more correctly, your "self" awareness merged with *the image* in your mind of your dream car. That is why it *felt* like the door hit you. It's as if you were your car.

But this identification took place only in your mind. This is easy to see here because the car you identified with was not even a real car. It is clear that you are not your imagined dream car. However, the identification makes it possible for you to feel emotional and physical sensations associated with the mental construct of the woman's car door hitting yours.

Here is the power imagination. If we identify with anything; even a belief, an idea or image of something in our mind, we will feel and react to what happens to the object of our identification as if it was personal and it happened to us in reality. This is no different than what occurs when we are watching a really good movie where we lose all sense of our "self". Once identified with the character or situation in the movie, it feels like we are the character and our body simply reacts to this idea believing it to be true!

Please note: any unpleasant reactions you felt when that car door hit your imaginary car were triggered by this perception in your mind. Nothing and no one was really hit, but we all have had experiences of how it feels to be hit and we project these feelings to the car because of our identification with it.

Clearly, we cannot be that which *belongs* to us, physical or non-physical. We can only imagine that we are them, projecting past feeling we have felt, onto them. Things cannot feel. Only living beings have emotional reactions and these reactions come from what we believe to be true in our perceiving mind.

Pay attention to the language you use to describe a past event, a car accident perhaps. The facts are: two cars collide; one is driven by you and the other by someone else. Notice the identification when you explain the event, "I (identification) was making a turn and out of nowhere this guy (identification of the driver with their car) hit me (identification)!" This interpretation makes the auto collision quite personal.

We can be really hard and unforgiving with others and our "self" when we don't understand that it is the identification that is making things feel so personal. We can come to believe that we, or others, are the cause of our hurtful reactions and come to blame ourselves or them for our pain. Yet, it is possible to be responsible and hold others accountable for words and behavior, without needing to make it personal and needing to assign blame.

When we are identifying with things that can get damaged or self-made images that can get devalued, we can't help but feel hurt. We are seeing and believing our "self" to be a thing that is vulnerable to deterioration and damage, affected by people's judgments and behaviors. But take away the identification, and we open our mind to seeing things more objectively and perhaps noticing an observing presence that senses itself as the stage on which all events unfold in our life and the one containing all that we possess.

If you can notice when you are identified and taking something personally, you can learn to see and understand errors differently. The problem is not with us or others, but with our thinking and our identifications. Our dream car's side getting hit would not have caused us emotional suffering without our identification. Any damage to a physical car would need repairing, but the feelings of personal hurt and attack need not necessarily be there.

Everything we make, imaginary or physical, is not eternal. To acquire a thing expecting that it will never deteriorate is to set our "self" up for future experiences of disappointment and loss. To identify our "self" with temporary things subject to decay is to accept a false identity and suffer the grief that comes when they are damaged or lost.

What needs to be recognized is how often we identify with our thinking and our things, including our body, and how much suffering this brings us. The great news is that we can correct our misperceptions and let go of our misidentifications by the practice of observing our perceiving mind. This will help us to respond to situations the way we really want to and not just helplessly react, driven by the emotional pain triggered by our interpretations and identifications. We will be able to see with more clarity and take things less personally. This will help us feel good about our "self" and others.

With desire and persistence we will be able to watch our thinking and notice our reactions coming not from us, but from the database of information in our perceiving mind. When we see ourselves and others making mistakes, we'll be more forgiving and ready to change how we are seeing the situation and the underlying beliefs. This understanding will shine rays of positive light on the way we see and value our "self" and others.

I hope that you are beginning to see that it may be in your best interests to choose to stop believing that the thinking mind is a savior, though it is quite useful to us. I want to open up your perceiving mind to the possibility of trusting and following what works beyond our thinking: inner wisdom, Higher Self, Holy Spirit, Christ Mind etc., however your spiritual beliefs have label it.

Chapter 9: Choice in Listening to Our Thinking

Is it possible to have a choice on whether not to just question our thinking, but also to decide NOT to listen to it? Perhaps to many of us this possibility sounds absurd and unsafe. After all, we don't want to disregard our parent's advice on the importance of thinking before acting. What our parents did not understand is that the lesson of thinking before acting, taken too seriously, closes us to listening to our intuition. If we listen to ALL our thinking, positive AND negative, we may be led into problems, rather than away from them.

If we listen to our negative "self" images, we are only reinforcing them and making them more real to us. If we listen to our fearful thoughts, we will be looking for what we want to avoid, increasing the chance of finding that. If we listen to our survival beliefs when there is no real physical threat, our primitive mind takes control when it doesn't need to, and we can easily misinterpret the situation, overreacting or keeping us from thinking clearly.

In not listening, I am not saying to deny or pretend that negative thoughts and emotions are not there. We still need to observe them. I'm saying, when they show up, they need acknowledgment but not belief. If we pay attention to their message because we believe it is the truth, we reinforce the negative thought patterns that gave rise to it. Because most often the negative thinking is subconscious, the best we can do is to become aware of the resulting negative emotions and allow them safe release so they stop anchoring the negative thinking.

When we suppress or ignore our emotions, we lose an important connection to uncovering those negative beliefs that are not serving us well and need correcting. Observing our mind's thinking and emotions brings us the awareness to begin correcting our problems. Without it, we live unconscious lives, following our subconscious database programming. We can't exercise conscious control in our life because we don't see we have a choice.

Identification keeps us stuck in unconscious mental, emotional and behavioral patterns that can falsely define what (who) we are. For this reason practicing meditation, yoga, Tai Chi, EFT (Emotional Freedom Techniques) or anything else mindfully and with persistence, can help retrain our attention and keep us from identifying with our thoughts, feelings, physical sensations, objects, etc. and be able to observe these without attachment or judgment.

This part of our mind that has the power to observe is our Higher Self, also referred to as the Higher Mind. We say it is "higher" because it can observe the "lower" perceiving mind at work: thinking, interpreting, analyzing, judging, distorting, etc., objectively and lovingly.

We really do have a choice whether to listen to our negative thinking or not! If we can catch it while it is happening, and even afterwards, we can come to decide what we want to do about it! We can choose to not believe what it is saying and choose another possibility for seeing things. We can take control of what has appeared to be an automatic process in our mind.

If we don't like what our negative interpretations are telling us about our "self", others and the world, we can look for a better perspective on how to see things. But our observation skills need to be practiced and developed, since the habit of automatically giving our attention and belief to all thought that show up is deeply engrained. Our negative reactions witness to this.

In my parenting role, I can recall when I allowed my own frustration and anger to speak through me to my children. Old wounds got stirred up by the situation with a child, and I lost control. As children, we often lacked understanding and the resources to help us work through the hurt we felt when our parents raised their voice and implied, "What is wrong with you!"

Unfortunately, many of us as children incorrectly concluded from these experiences, "I am the cause of the emotional upset that my mother/father is expressing." Similarly, we assumed that others were the cause of our emotional hurt. And yes, it did appear that way. But then we started noticing that it was not the other person directly causing the hurt, it felt like an invisible button got pushed and then our upset erupted.

What we were unaware of was the existence of our powerful database interpreters standing in between our interactions and communications with each other. How skillful and unbiased are our interpreters really? Do we walk away feeling misunderstood or frustrated that we did not communicate clearly?

While our behaviors or words may have been the trigger that set off the reaction in another person, we are all still responsible for both our reactions and actions and no one else. There is no blame. Remember what is directing our reactions? It is our less than completely accurate interpretations. Blame only supports further the misperceptions. Only by not identifying with our interpretations and seeing where they may not be true, can we begin to communicate fully.

We want to embrace responsibility for what is in our subconscious database because this is how we recognize we have the power to make the changes needed. Blame only serves to obscure this recognition because it places the cause of our suffering outside of ourselves, turning us into powerless victims in our mind.

When we leave blame out of the picture, we can see the good news that comes from realizing that our interpretations dictate our reactions. While we can't control other people's actions and words, we have the power to change our interpretation of those actions and words, and in turn, change our resulting feelings to give us more options for responding as we really want to.

This is great news because it means we are in charge of how we feel. The responsibility of how we feel rests with our thinking and our thinking is not outside of our control. Also, we can let go of guilt coming from the belief that we are to blame for other's (adults) upsets.

This does not relieve us of the responsibility we have for our behavior, but most of the time, people's emotional hurts are the result of misinterpretation, when in fact, there was no hurt intended. In other words, nothing personal was intended, but identification made it appear that way.

Unkind things may be said and done, but the question is, do we want to keep making those things personal to us and suffer as a result? People can say many "mean" things to each other, do we want to keep believing and reacting to negativity as if it was Truth? But even if we do want to believe that negativity as truth, does it change reality? No. Again, truth is truth and reality is reality. Any distortion of the truth happens only in the perceiving mind.

We must begin to observe our thinking if we want to ultimately catch our negative reactions before they take place. It takes our full willingness and compassionate practice to take charge of our subconscious processes, but it can be done.

Start questioning how you are seeing a situation when you begin to feel negativity stirring. Is there another way of interpreting what is going on that is more positive? Your interpretation determines whether you see a choice in how to respond. Do you want your past database of negative thinking and old wounds to keep speaking and controlling your behavior in new situations?

With "self" awareness of how perception works in our mind, we can begin to see more solutions. Maybe we can catch our perceiving mind when its thinking takes a turn for the worse and stop it before it takes us down a road we will later regret. We need to take charge of our thinking!

Use any stress reducing technique to help you pause before you react. Remember that many of your foundational negative conclusions are coming from the perceiving mind of a very young child who was doing the best he/she could do at that time.

Let go of judging your negative reactions "childish" or "foolish" because they are coming from the perspective of a hurt young child. It is time to bring understanding to the child's pain. This is how we open our hurts to healing and forgiving. This is how we grow and evolve through life.

Sometimes all we need to do is catch our mind thinking negatively and observe it without judgment, to bring about a deep change in perception. *Here is an example:*

I was at the hardware store early one day and ran into an acquaintance that I had not seen for a while. Later as I was making dinner, I caught my mind remembering an unflattering conversation I had overheard about this acquaintance, a few months back. The comments from my co-workers were about her children and some unpaid bills. As I observed this thinking, I noticed the energy of disapproval and negative value judgment. This was interesting. I wondered, "Out of all the memories my mind could be thinking about, why did it decide, out of my awareness, to bring up this particular one?"

As I considered this, I got the feeling that a part of my mind seemed to be feeding off the negative energy around the comments, relishing the put downs and literally sucking the family members of their goodness and self-esteem. I tuned in to this part of my mind that seemed to feel nourished by their demise, and in a second, it vanished completely. In its place, a completely opposite picture arose. I saw the mom and kids and felt deep compassion and love for them. I recognized that given their circumstances, like all of us, they were just doing their best trying to keep up with paying bills. Their inherent self-worth and goodness was self-evident and unquestionable.

In this experience, I saw how a part of my mind holds onto negative comments and judgments, much like a dog that buries bones to dig up later and leisurely chew on them. You can almost say that our perceiving mind develops a habit for feeding off negativity, if we don't keep an eye on it.

Perhaps I could not help overhearing the comments my co-workers made about this acquaintance. In that moment, I lacked the awareness to question the negativity implied in their words and I accepted the comments as true. But, if I can catch this part of my mind thinking about the memory, I will then have a choice to observe it and change it. This is one way to open up negative memories to Truth and clear them from our subconscious database. It is a step towards regaining control of our negative perceiving mind, and by extension, changing how we see our "self" and others.

Again, be conscious of the information you are exposing your perceiving mind to. Information is energy and our database will *feed on* it. Whether it is your co-workers gossiping, or what you are doing for entertainment. Notice the type of beliefs and perceptions that your habits are nourishing. Do you really want to listen to images and words that support existing negative views or fears that trigger your mind-body into survival mode?

The recognition that we have a choice in what to believe and give our attention to in our thinking, gives us immense power in influencing the type of experiences we have and their impact on our life. This is because our world of experiences acts like a mirror, reflecting back to us the information in our database, through our reactions and interpretations.

Our inner and outer worlds are not separate. In choosing how we want to interpret something, we are choosing how we want to feel and how we will perceive our life! This is a self-reinforcing pattern: our interpretations give rise to our emotions; our emotions drive our reactions; our reactions give our current experience its meaning; and this meaning is interpreted by our perceiving mind as validation for how true its existing beliefs are; the existing beliefs get stronger and filter out what we see in our new experiences to match them; this introduces bias in our interpretations, which then give rise to our emotions and so on.

We often say, "He *made me* so angry!" Did someone wave a magic wand and turn us into anger? Can someone force us to feel the emotion of anger if we don't want to? No;

but it is difficult not to identify with our feelings and see that our "self" is not the anger we are feeling. It is also difficult not to react with anger when something has triggered it from within us without practicing self-awareness.

Due to our strong identification with our emotions, we can come to fear them and may opt to suppress them to feel safe or in control. Often we judge them bad, a sign of weakness, or seeing no point to them, prefer to hide or cut-off their expression. Emotions vibrate so strongly and deeply in our body that it takes much effort to make believe they are not there. Anger flushes our face with heat, fear tightens our chest or stomach, sadness brings up tears, etc. What we may do then, is disconnect from our feelings all together.

Here is an example **from** *my life:*

My first semester in college I began questioning my choice of majors and was feeling very confused. I was talking to a professor about this, and she suggested that I think back to the moments in my life when I was the most happy to get insight into what field of work I might enjoy.

I tried this and looked back to find those happy memories. To my surprise I could not find any! This was disturbing to me because I didn't feel unhappy about my life either. I grew up knowing my parents loved me and had given me the best they could. I had friends and excelled in school and was very active in clubs, sports and my church. I wondered, "How could I not have been happy, at least some times? "

What finally dawned on me from this experience was that I had disconnected myself from my feelings. At an early age I had concluded that how I felt did not matter to what was happening in my life. So, I stopped paying attention to how I felt. I could not find any happy memories because the feelings had not been consciously acknowledged in the moment of the experience and made a part of the memory.

For the child, this strategy of disconnecting from her feelings solved the problem of having to deal with difficult negative emotions. Unfortunately, disconnecting from our feelings is an all or nothing deal. Feelings are feelings, regardless of whether they are positive or negative. If we don't want to feel the negative ones, we won't be able to connect to the positive ones either.

When I realized this, I started paying attention to my feelings again. It took a while for me to relearn how to connect to what I felt inside and name it correctly, but with practice, I did it.

Emotions play a very important part in anchoring our interpretations to physical reality by the associated bodily sensations they produce. When we feel our emotions vibrating like the sound of guitar strings being plucked and amplified by a hollow body, it is hard to deny what they are saying. This is why some of us take drastic measures when we don't want to hear their tune.

What we can now realize is that we don't need to cut off our feelings to get relief from them or to feel in control, all we need to do is change how we see the situation, and this changes the associated emotional and physical effects.

Let me demonstrate the power of this idea with an example:

When I was just beginning to practice EFT, I was watching a DVD of a workshop given by a Master EFT Practitioner. As I noticed how incredibly knowledgeable and helpful he was, I began to feel down and deflated. I felt like I might as well give up my practice and crawl under a rock because he knew so much more than me. I was ready to go lie down because I had lost all my energy and felt so tired. But I stopped and noticed these feelings, and wondered why I felt like that?

So, I retraced my thoughts. I observed what my mind did. It compared my EFT Certification Level 1 "self" to this EFT Master "self" and concluded that I was NOT *measuring up* in a BIG way. I recognized that my perceiving mind had reached this conclusion automatically, as if by habit. It occurred to me however, that my perceiving mind could have reached a different conclusion.

It could have admired the Master's talents and appreciated how willing he was to share his expertise. This would then make me feel grateful for the opportunity to learn from him. I would also feel motivated to improve my own skills and abilities. By running this alternative choice of perspective through my mind, it changed how I felt immediately. I felt great, excited and full of energy.

This is the power of interpretation. Within a couple of minutes I went from feeling deflated and giving up on my EFT Practice, to feeling excited and looking forward to growing and moving ahead.

Chapter 10: What is True and What is Truth

I have attempted to show you where our thinking and perception is distorting truth and reality so that you will question and not believe the negative interpretations of your "self". The ultimate goal of this book is to help you recognize the Truth of your identify and connect to the part of your mind that resonates to this Truth.

When our perceptions and interpretations are saying negative things and we indulge them with our belief and feel their associated negative emotions, we are strengthening their energy and making then truer in our perceiving mind. Just because we can believe and feel quite sure something negative is true about us, it may not be that way at all, if we were to look at it from a different angle. Remember my EFT Master DVD example.

All positive and negative beliefs and feelings reside in the perceiving part of our mind. However, only positive, uplifting and unconditionally loving ones support Truth. That's why deep soulful feelings, like those that arise when looking at the amazing beauty of nature, fill us with positive energy and peace. Truth cannot be the cause of our self-esteem problems because those negative perceptions deflate us, weigh us down and belittle us. Truth enlivens, uplifts, fills us with Spirit and life giving energy.

When we feel bad about our "self", it means we are holding a belief that appears to be true, but is not in Truth. Truth, with a "th", refers to Spiritual Truth. It resides at the spiritual level beyond perception and cannot be changed by perception. The closest we can come to Truth with our dirty water filters is to clean out the negativity and choose to believe in the complete purity of our life. This requires that we trust wholeheartedly that only good things are possible because our Creator is without a doubt, unconditionally loving. Trusting in this aligns our perceiving mind to to seek only goodness, and it will then find it.

You may be thinking, "This is easier said than done!" Yes, it can appear that way. Because I work with clients whose experiences of trauma speak to them as reliable witnesses to the impossibility of this idea, I understand the resistance. But, once the negative energy is released from the memories of the traumas, perception is free to see things in a better light. We all have a Higher Mind that recognizes and desires only Truth.

Thomas Jefferson, the writer of the USA Declaration of Independence, recognized Truth and referred to it when he stated, *"We hold these truths to be self-evident, that all men are created equal, that they are endowed by their Creator with certain unalienable Rights, that among these are Life, Liberty and the pursuit of Happiness."*

I am interpreting this as saying: without exception all people are created equal, they all have divine rights that cannot be taken away such as life, liberty and the pursuit of happiness. He was writing about divine Truth, with a "th". Spiritual Truth does not exclude anyone. Though Mr. Jefferson used the term "men", I believe he was including everyone regardless of gender, economic status, age, color, etc. precisely because he was speaking about universal Truth.

He also says, "We hold these truths to be *self-evident...*" because he recognized that Truth does not reside at the level of belief or perception. Our Higher Mind recognizes Truth and so it is "self-evident".

Truth cannot come to us by way of our thinking mind. If it did, it would get distorted as it passed by the filters of our existing foundational beliefs so it would match and support them. Mr. Jefferson was not saying, "Think, analyze and consider these ideas and you may come to agree with me." He is speaking directly to our Higher Mind, attempting to bypass the filters of our perceptual database that cannot know truth, but only *thinks* it can.

Our Higher Mind, like the well that gives us access to the pure water from the deeper Source, is our connection to Truth and bypasses the plumbing and faucet filter altogether. Truth *resonates* or *rings* true within us because our perceptual database is not involved and we simply recognize its pure taste. For these reasons, Truth is above and beyond our perception.

Truth, however, is not beyond our experience and recognition, as long as we keep our perceiving mind open and *want* to hear the Truth, and nothing else. If not, we will run the Truth we hear through our perceiving mind, putting what is pure water through a dirty filter. But remember that the filtering process cannot do away with Truth, though it distorts it in our mind's eye, keeping us stuck experiencing polluted interpretations.

Another way to describe the recognition of Truth is that it gives us an "Aha" moment. It brings deep insight and understanding. For me, such insights leave certainty. Some people refer to this as a knowing. We all have the ability to open up and receive Truth. The knowing is the recognition of it. But again, we need to value Truth above perception.

This means letting go of our identification to our perceptions, to being always "right" and understanding that our database will be "wrong" more often than we care to admit. This is the humility that is needed for our mind to open up and accept Truth. When Truth is embraced, our perceiving mind is automatically corrected and contradictory beliefs released.

Choosing to open our mind to Truth despite fears and appearances opens up new possibilities for how we can value and know our "self". When we observe that our perceiving mind has reached its limits and has no answers for us, we have a window of opportunity to turn our ears and listen to the inner wisdom of our Higher Mind through the love in our heart. We can go beyond our thinking mind and connect with the spiritual dimension where our true "Self" resides.

Because we have unconsciously given our perceiving mind so much control over our life, it will resist change. This part of our mind often perceives Truth as a threat and will defend its beliefs with a fervent zeal, distorting reality in the process as necessary.

Here is another example of how easy it is to hide and guard our misperceptions:

I had picked up a large order of food for dinner, which included five drinks. I had everything fairly secure on a lid from a cardboard box and I just needed to put it in my car. I was in a hurry (survival mode for me), and the thought to put the food on the back seat of the car occurred to me. I didn't question this thought, despite other information that pointed out that it would be better placed on the floor, since the drinks could spill and the mess would end up on the seat. But, I did not listen to this information. True to this premonition, one of the lemonades tipped over drenching the back seat.

While driving my car the next morning, I reflected on the lemonade spill and that for some reason, I had disregarded what was clearly helpful advice from my intuition. This brought up a memory of another very similar incident that had taken place a month or so in the past.

I was also in a hurry and didn't have time to finish my lunch. My sandwich was so good, I decided to take it with me and eat it while driving. Immediately after this decision, I recall receiving distinct information showing me a scene where the half sandwich was sliding off my plate and falling all over my lap and the car interior. Did I listen? No. And sure enough, that sandwich slid right off my plate the moment I opened the car door and started to get in the car.

So that morning I couldn't help but wonder, "Is there is something important for me to learn here that I am obviously not seeing? Why is this situation repeating?" I decided to use EFT tapping to see what insights I might receive.

I started by tuning into the lemonade spill event, observing my thoughts and feelings as I was getting ready to put the food in the car. I sensed that the decision to put the drinks in the back seat was automatic and locked in. I guessed, "Maybe I have an automatic pilot for decision making and it turns on when I'm in a hurry?"

I tuned into the "locked in" feeling. I felt an unwillingness to consider other options from this part of my mind. It was turning a deaf ear to my intuition. It did not want its decision questioned. I wondered, "Why not? What if I did question the decision, what would that mean to this part of my mind?" The feeling that came as I considered this question was that accepting information from my intuition meant this part of my mind was accepting correction and that meant... admitting it was wrong!

Aha! This part of my mind felt it was being corrected by my intuition and did not like it. I continued questioning, "Why not? What is wrong with being wrong?" I tuned into the feeling of "not liking it when I am wrong". I noticed an underlying conclusion that said, "There is something wrong with me (identification) when I (identification) make a mistake." This felt bad.

Without the mess in the car and without questioning my thinking mind, I would not have found the negative "self" image and identification underlying the mess. Now this negative view can be cleared because it is not the Truth. I am not my mistakes, nor am I the part of my mind that fears correction.

What we see here is that emotional pain looks for attention and a way out. I can see how those car messes were just reflecting the underlying belief, "There must be something wrong with me; look at this mess!" The outer reflects the inner. Let's choose to reflect Truth instead of negative misperceptions and stop needing to make a mess to get our attention.

From my perspective, our sacred work on earth is to bring healing to our mind's misperceptions so they can come into alignment with the Truth of our Higher Mind. Any situation, belief or misperception that carries negativity or hurt is calling for our understanding and attention so that it can heal.

Chapter 11: Self-images and Labels

Children growing up in the Western world are introduced to an idea that says they have to become *somebody* when they grow up. We are also given a message that says, "You have a life, now go and make *something* out of it."

What are these ideas implying? If we have to become *somebody* or make *something* of our life, then, are we inherently *nobody* and our life *nothing* and worthless until we do?

Let's explore the implications. If the child needs to turn her/his "self" into *something* or *someone*, then what the child is without doing this, must by default, be incomplete or not enough to start with. Otherwise, there would be no need to improve, or make the "self" into *somebody* or *something* else. It also implies that what the child *does* or *accomplishes* in the betterment of their "self" is what gives them value.

This perspective assumes that the "self" starts out in life like a blob of clay that needs sculpturing to define it and make it into *something* beautiful and valuable. If this is not done, the "self" is seen as a *nothing*. Look around: is there any other form of life that starts out as *nothing* to become *something* else? No. Can any living thing not be its "self" from the start? A Redwood Tree starts out as a Redwood Tree. A dog starts out as a little dog, called a puppy. Even a Monarch Butterfly that starts out as a caterpillar is still a butterfly before it goes through its metamorphosis. Otherwise, the caterpillar would never turn into a butterfly and they would be two separate insects.

Along a similar line, how many times have we asked a child, "What are you going to *be* when you grow up?" Perhaps what we really meant to say was, "What are you going to *do* when you grow up?" We have inadvertently made *doing* and *being* the same. Is picking out a career picking out what we are? Would we not be the same person regardless of a change in jobs? This misunderstanding makes it easy for us to identify with what we do, our behavior or work.

Through identification, it does appear as if we are what we do. Unfortunately, social values and conventions have determined that all doing is not equal and so, different work pays different wages. For many individuals that are identified with their jobs this translates into: working in a lower paying job or not having a job means, "I am less valuable."

Clearly it is easy to have our self regard tied to the perceived worth of our work or net worth. To see our "self" as what we do or what we earn is a type of self-image identification. This belief of identity in the form of an image is in our mind's eye only. A self-image of us is made, a nurse for example, and is then used to compare our current "self" as a nurse to the ideal image nurse that is the standard for measurement. The ideal self-image contains a definition of how a "nurse" should be. We use this to compare our "self" and judge our relative performance and value with respect to the ideal. This is how we evaluate how well we have sculptured our "self" to the desired mold provided by the ideal self-image. We compare to see how close we have come to making our "self" into that valuable something.

Identification with the self-image of the "something" or "somebody" we should be or want to be makes the idea of self-esteem possible. Self-esteem becomes the feeling of pride that indicates our success in accomplishing the ideal standard self-image. Only comparison can tell us if we have become that *somebody* and can feel valuable. This works fine as long as our perceiving mind sees success.

However, self-identity and self-esteem is lost when our efforts don't measure up to the requirements of our self-image definitions and identifications. If we have identified with our job and lose it, it follows that without it, we are *nothing*. Our identity, our job, has gone and we have nothing in its place, or what we do have is not good enough. From this perspective, our sense of "self" and value got taken away with our job.

Or perhaps we did something in our life that we are not proud of. If we are what we do and if we can't feel proud of what we did, how can we have self-esteem when pride is the essential element? So, we need to question this part of our mind that accepts and makes up definitions. Are we really what we do? How can one aspect of how we engage in life be us?

Are we not ourselves when we are relaxing, sleeping or just observing the present moment without doing anything?

By insisting on seeing our "self" as what we do, we can expect that our value will fluctuate by changes to our doing and by negative criticism or judgment of our work. Identifying with a self-image and fluctuating self-esteem go hand-in-hand.

All the "I am" labels we accept as our identity like: I am a student; I am an architect; I am a mother; I am a father; I am helpful; and I am vulnerable, etc. are labels of identification of our "self". They are predefined self-images. The "self" image swallows-up our consciousness for as long as the identification lasts. In this state of identification we believe we are the self-image in our perceiving mind. It is like playing a character in a play and then getting stuck with the mask we put on, forgetting we are only pretending to be the mask and believing it is what we are.

The ability to observe our thinking is lost when we try to fit our "self" into a mold defined by a self-image. We are then trying to be something we are not, reacting to any negative criticism of these self-images as personal attacks. Since we are identified, we can't see that our "self" is not the one getting put-down, only the self-image of our "self", and so, we feel its hurt.

Here is a made up example to illustrate this point:

A parent comes to school and complains to her child's teacher that the homework she gave was very confusing and the child could not do it. The teacher could take this personally, feeling criticized and devalued. She could dwell on it and feed the thoughts that are saying, "You are not a very good teacher." But she doesn't need to take this route.

If she can recognize she is not her work and that the parent's interpretation of the homework is not necessarily truth, she can see the information coming to her more objectively. Seeing that she is not her work does not mean that the teacher will disregard the parent's comments. The complaint becomes just information, neither good nor bad, and can be used to see if her lesson needs revision. She will look for more information and ask the rest of the kids in class how they found the homework. If more kids found it confusing, she will see that the homework needs revising, or she needs to spend more time teaching the concepts to the whole class, or perhaps just the parent's child. The teacher learns and grows from this experience benefitting everyone.

All "self" images and identifications exist only in our mind and reflect a belief that our "self" is not completely acceptable as it is. They are representations of what we have come to *believe* and *think* we should be, have been, or are; and what we *see, feel* or *want* our "self" to be. We do not know our essential "Self" and therefore, have accepted the idea that it is partly or entirely worthless. And so, we strive and struggle to earn our worth by making this lowly "self" into some*thing* or some*body* of valuable.

Self-images cannot fill our longing for certainty, wholeness and deep fulfillment. For this reason our perceiving mind is quite desperate and easily accepts and seeks identification with labels and just about anything and everything, without regard for how they make us feel. It can identify with the new designer shoes that we just bought, or with the cold sore on the side our mouth that just showed up. Either way, we will feel self-image conscious.

Our deeper and more stable self-images often come from how others have seen us and from the names they called us when we were little. Sometimes they arise from our own conclusions, interpretation and names we have called our "self".

We may say and think, "I am intelligent; I am beautiful; I am weak; I am stupid; I am a good parent; I am disrespected; I am a hypocrite; I am financially secure; I am a looser; I am a mechanic; I am a war veteran or I am a sinner." The list goes on and on. It does not matter whether these are positive or negative; they are all identifications and subjective assessments based on accepted definitions believed to be true.

This is why perceiving our "self" as our behaviors, actions, choices, occupation, physical traits, personal preferences, etc. limits us to some *thing* and can only give us an incomplete, confusing and fragmented picture of what we are.

Our consciousness can only be identified with one *thing* at a time. You may have noticed that you can hold contradictory beliefs about your "self". You can believe you are smart in some things and stupid in others. This is possible because our self-images do not integrate into one whole being, they remain separate and apart, and that is how we often feel when we are identified with a self-image, incomplete and separate.

I had a client who was struggling in college. A part of her problem was that she had grown up being called the Pretty One. Her younger sister got labeled the Smart One. But because she had accepted this image of the Pretty One as her "self", she felt very vulnerable and limited in an intellectual environment. She doubted her *smarts* because she did not see her "self" as intelligent. While there were advantages to seeing herself as the Pretty One and her sister as the Smart One, now she saw the limitations of the label and needed to change her perceiving mind in this regard.

Unaware of our wholeness and true identity, we easily identify with labels and self-images. This approach to knowing our "self" is so pervasive that we rarely question whether we can really know our "self" with the perceiving part of our mind. Once we label something by giving it a name, we think we know its identity; when really, it is only a limited description of words and beliefs that perhaps others agree with.

Without questioning our beliefs, we teach what has been passed down to us. Our children then accept the perceptual distortions in these beliefs if they don't question them, passing them on generationally.

I recall my daughter asking me a fundamental question of identity at age four: "Am I going to die?" Unfortunately, I did not recognize the spiritual nature of this question and said, "Yes honey, we all die." I believed I was speaking the truth, but I was identified and only speaking about the body.

Upon hearing my answer, she looked devastated and broke down crying. Honestly, I felt terrible, but I did not know what else to say. In retrospect, I would've liked to have said, "No honey. You are a part of Life and Life cannot die; only bodies die. Life never dies."

Maybe some of you are saying, "That is also a belief." Yes it is, and a very powerful one because it is about our identity. And in my heart, I would much rather support an identity belief that is boundless, eternal and fearless; rather than one that is limited, fragile and born just to die.

But alas, I could only give her what I believed then. And in the end, it is all fine anyway. Our beliefs do not make or change Truth. When our perceiving mind tries to change

Truth, as in my *Toy Story III* example, we simply lose sight of it, but we haven't changed it.

I see that it is in my best interests to want to correct my beliefs so they support spiritual Truth, in this way I will not hide them from my "self". But we don't need to worry that our perceptual distortions affect reality in any way, because they don't. What we need to notice is the immense power our beliefs have on how we experience life.

When we change our beliefs, we are changing how we see (interpret) our experiences and therefore, the quality of the experience, not the facts of the experience. Don't underestimate the power of your beliefs, especially your self-images. They will match the quality of your life experiences.

My daughter, like all of us, is given all the time in the world and all the opportunities necessary to understand and accept responsibility for this amazing power. When she is ready, she will want to let go of any negative beliefs she accepted from her parents that are no longer serving her life experience well.

With regard to self-images as labels, when my son was a toddler I would take him to the park at the school where I volunteered. He would play nearby while I chatted with other adults who would ask, "How old is your son? Is he ready for Kindergarten?

When I answered that he was only three years old, they would often reply in amazement, "He is a *big guy*!" And I would agree because he was tall for his age. But I had no idea my playing toddler had been listening and making conclusions about his identity. One day, however, he surprised me when I said, "Come on Oscar, get in the car." He replied very assertively, "Me not Oscar, me Big Guy!"

We learn to identify very early with names and labels and many stay with us for a lifetime. I have worked with clients that have continued to identify with strong negative labels they heard as children such as "troubled child", or even words they heard in the womb like, "unwanted baby".

These labels are also used by our perceiving mind to focus our attention on finding matching information in new situations. Our behavior will follow instructions from these deeply ingrained, programmed self-images. If we believe our program that dictates we are a "loser", we will convey its decree in our lives. It will act like a model for our behavior to imitate. The negative self-image will be used unconsciously like a map to follow in new situations, reinforcing itself with our behavior in the process.

But thank goodness these "self" images and our identifications exist only at the perception level. It means they can change and do. How we saw our "self" at age five is much different than the way we see our "self" now. Some things perhaps seem to have stayed the same, but we would all say we are quite different now. We went through many changes, and this helped to modify the existing beliefs and perceptions we had of our "self", to what they are now. This reassures us that our negative images are not permanent and can be modified or let go of completely.

Variability in self-esteem is the result of changes in self-image identification. The fluctuation happens because specific emotions are associated with each particular self-perception we hold in the moment. Positive self-images make us feel good and valuable, and negative ones don't. Which of your many "self" images are you identified with when instead of feeling pride, you feel shame or unworthiness?

Here is an example of how easily we can lower our self-esteem through identification:

Just before our third child was born, I decided to be (identification) a stay-at-home mom (negative self-image). I did it because I wanted to be (identification) a good parent (positive self-image) and felt it was too hard to accomplish this working a full time job. Unfortunately for this good parent image that I desire to be, I was unable to consistently get my kids to school on time even as a stay-at-home mom (identification).

This produced anger directed at my son when I waited for him in the car in the mornings. It felt like each time I failed to get him there on time, it said something negative about me. So of course I would get angry at him!

From the perspective of the "self" that wanted to be a good parent, I had done my motherly duty by packing my son's lunch, making him breakfast and waiting in the car to go. It seemed like it was my son's lack of attention to the clock that kept me from achieving what I wanted: to become a good parent. Given this interpretation, I felt justified in making my son the problem and being angry with him.

In looking at this experience, I noticed that the decision to be a *good parent* was mine, and I could not have made it without consulting my subconscious database for the definition of *"good parent"*. Otherwise, how could I have decided it was a good idea to strive to be that in the first place?

Part of my definition had to include something like, "Not getting your kids to school on time excludes you from being a *good parent*." Also, notice my definition did not say anything about making my child responsible for my anger, so that was fine from my point of view. But, my son was not the cause of the anger I felt. It came from my definition because it excluded me from what I wanted to be. This brought up a doubt and fear that this meant I was a *bad parent* instead.

Here is the point I want to make. Regardless of the definition of *good parent* that I had and how I acquired it, it was still my definition. I could have questioned it and modified it so I could have felt better about my "self". In practice, however, this was not possible. The problem was: I identified with trying to be a *good parent* and could not observe my thinking to understand where my reactions where really coming from. I was left unconscious, without a choice to see things differently and without self-esteem, since my identification with being a stay-at-home mom was negative. I could not feel good about my "self ", doubting I was a *good parent* and fearing I was a *bad parent.*

Could my inconsistency in getting my child to school on time really exclude me from being a *good parent* or worse, turn me into a *bad parent*? Only my identification to the definition of *good parent* could lead me to believe that this was true, since I failed to meet its criteria. In wanting to make my "self" into a *good parent,* I set up the possibility of failing to fit this mold and opened up the possibility of making my "self" into a *bad parent* instead. Of course this situation was upsetting, but not for the reasons I thought.

We lose our power to change and see things differently when we don't recognize that it is the definitions and identifications we hold that give rise to our negative feelings that bring down our self-esteem. We cannot make a choice we do not recognize we have, nor exercise power to change our life when we believe we are victims of our external circumstances, or of other people.

Most of us go through life not understanding that through perception we can redefine how we see our "self" and our life, and that this brings about the external changes we want. Again, my self-images, identifications and definitions kept my consciousness stuck and limited to seeing my son as the cause for my upset, and my "self" as a failure.

When our self-image definitions are unrealistic in what we are trying to *be,* they can easily turn negative on us. Success coaches understand this and emphasize setting achievable goals, ones that the client can be sure to reach. The last thing they want to see happen is for their client to end up reinforcing a perception of failure, if the goal is not reached.

The bottom line is, as adults we have the power to choose how to see our "self". We are the ones that accept and keep the labels and definitions of our self-images. Though many of these lay hidden in our subconscious, we do see their reflections in our life.

There is no need to judge the reflections. They are just information to be used for updating our databases and for growth. They are windows into our subconscious database and opportunities to learn what we are NOT, and perhaps, even that our true value is found beyond these beliefs and self-images.

Let me restate what I learned from the school situation. It was not my son, nor his behavior, nor the fact that I could not consistently get him to school on time that caused my upset and low self-esteem. It was identification and the desire to turn my "self" into the self-image of what I believed a *good parent* should be. My failure to meet its definition conditions implied that I might be a *bad parent* instead, which felt upsetting and "self" devaluating.

Through identification with my self-images, I delegate power to my database to measure and decide my worth. However, my database cannot know me in Truth. It can only measure the worth of self-images. My perceiving mind cannot see beyond its own stored data. I can never know my true essential "Self" through my thinking. That Truth becomes self-evident as I learn to connect more to intuitive guidance from my Higher Mind.

Chapter 12: Survival and Self-images

Self-esteem issues for many of us involve defending or proving our "self". It can feel like our value is in danger of being taken away and needs defending; or is not apparent and needs proving to others. Striving to prove our "self" can turn into a matter of survival.

For some of my clients who grew up with a family story of feeling consistently ignored, put-down, blamed, unrecognized, unloved or perhaps hated, self-esteem took second place to feeling safe. Making their "self" into a self-image that got approval became of the highest priority, because it felt like it would protect them from attack.

These clients learned to equate approval with survival. Disapproval became a sign for danger. From this perspective, controlling how others saw and reacted to them became their number one priority in their social interactions. For good reason, they felt safer alone, though they felt isolated and longed for companionship.

To these clients, interacting with someone that was upset was like having a dangerous lions roaring in front of their face. Understandably, they identified with their fears and had a difficult time seeing that people's upsets were not personal. Some were eager to please, others ready to defend and attack, and all strived to *be* perfect matches to self-image standards they believed came from the expectations of others.

We saw earlier the difficulty I had in trying to become the self-image called *"good parent"*. The problem for these clients went deeper since they needed a match to their model image to feel safe. They were trying to become who they *thought someone else* wanted them to be; trying to match their "self" to a self-image made from reading the expectations of others.

It would be like a chameleon that changes color to blend in with his environment to stay safe from predators. Only for these clients, the environment changed color sporadically and unexpectedly. The self-image, or color, the chameleon displayed would then be a mismatch to the changed environment. This made my clients feel visible, vulnerable and unsafe.

They were constantly trying to guess what would be pleasing to the other people in their life. They walked on eggshells hoping not to disturb the sleeping lion. Without a fixed definition to match their behavior to, failure was inevitable and their state of survival activated even more.

Their negative self-judgment for failing to measure up was very harsh and unforgiving, often matching the judgments they received as children. This only served to keep them stuck in a self-perpetuating cycle that increased fear, frustration and anxiety around others.

Whenever we feel our "self" to be in a situation of survival, we are identifying our "self" with an image that is weak and subject to pain and loss. Whatever the self-image we have identified with, it will be seen as vulnerable to being hurt. Our instinctive reactions of fight, flight or freeze kicks in.

The point I am making is that when our self-images get stuck in fear and survival, it is very difficult to let go of our identification. We need help. The problem is that survival mode disconnects us from our Higher Mind, and limits our ability to help ourselves. Our options get limited to fight, flee and freeze reactions.

I worked with an EFT client tapping on trauma she experienced. Metaphorically it felt like she had been abandoned in the middle of a desert without a sign of life anywhere. We brought resolution to the survival fears, but there was additional tapping to do to release the blame she assigned to her "self" for "Not trusting in God" during the traumatic time.

Our survival mind cannot trust in God. Putting trust in something beyond itself is not within its primitive abilities. We lose connection with our higher self-awareness in the moment we identify with survival. Fear takes charge of our perception. For this reason, it is a good idea to seek qualified help in these situations. It does not say anything negative about us when we do.

My client was upset that she did not turn to God during that intensely fearful and isolating time in her life. She interpreted her behavior as lacking in faith. But we all get stuck in survival mode from time to time, and it is not that we lack faith in God. We just don't see other options, especially those that are always available to us from our Higher Mind which connects with Spirit and infinite possibility.

I gave the example of my client above because I want to encourage compassion towards our "self" at all times. We need it most when we are scared and feeling as if our survival is threatened.

Chapter 13: Value and Worth

If you go to an electronics store and see a cool looking gadget but have no idea what it does, would you want to buy it? With the limited information you have, it would be difficult to determine if it has any value to you. Value implies importance and without more information, you don't know if it is important to you. We only want what is perceived as important, beneficial to us. The value of something is then determined by its perceived importance.

What determines what is important and beneficial to us? Definitions of value and importance also come from the beliefs that we acquired during our upbringing and learning. The beliefs represent what we have learned, deemed or judged to be important.

However, for many of us, our definitions of value do not distinguish between objects and people and apply value judgment equally to both. They attempt to assign value to human beings, like objects, based on the importance and usefulness in meeting our desires. When this part of our mind does this, it is seeing relationships as financial consumer transactions.

This part of our mind can come to believe that it has the power to give or take away value from our "self" and others, in the same way that it assigns value or devalues things it is considering purchasing. It makes a note of differences, compares and decides a person's worth based on how much benefit can be derived from them.

While this process of comparing and judging value works great when we shop, and helps to select what has the best value *for us*. It gradually sets precedence, like judicial law setting up standards for judging similar cases based on the conclusions of past similar ones. This precedence makes it easier to judge value quickly in new situations. It becomes a type of map or template in our database for comparing, rating, and categorizing by degrees. We can then judge: "This is best (good) and this, the opposite end, is worst (bad)"; quickly and with confidence that we are right.

This is what our preferences and likes are: templates for judging what has value to us. Anything we like has perceived value for us. Anything, and unfortunately by extension, anyone we dislike, doesn't have much.

When we identify with our preferences, we take them very personally. They can come to define a large part of our personality. They are the criteria, rules and definitions for quickly deciding such mundane things as: which type of tea or coffee do I want to drink? Which bag of bread should I buy? The template takes into consideration what is important to us in terms of taste, type, price, size, brand etc. We are looking for the best fit to what we like and will exclude what we don't like.

Which movie should we see? This question is run by our movie preference template. We take into account information about the type of movie, the actors in it, who invited us, where it is playing, the rating, etc. In choosing, it is about what has been established as important to us, but also the relative importance of the criteria. If we really like the person we are going to the movies with, in this case, it may not matter at all what movie we see! If we are seeing the movie by ourselves, we most likely would give more value to the type of movie, price, time, etc.

It's important to note, the value we assign to something is relative. It can feel like it is set in stone, but our preferences change with time, and they also depend on what is getting compared in the moment.

Here is an exercise for you to observe how your mind decides value:

Pay attention to how you select food at a buffet table or at a special event that has a varied selection. Stop and notice your mind's decision process. What thoughts cross your mind as you are choosing? What did you look for and consider? You will be surprised to notice how complex this choice is, or perhaps it will be quite simple.

In some areas of our life our preferences are stronger than in others, or sometimes we make exceptions. Perhaps you haven't eaten all day and don't care what food you eat now as long as it fills your empty stomach. The point is that our mind has been trained to compare, evaluate, judge and take into account what is important to us. It saves us time in making the many small, every-day decisions.

Identification with our likes and dislikes is what keeps us loyal to particular products when shopping. Though it helps us select what we want quickly at a large department or grocery store, it can close our mind to other options that could save us money. Nevertheless, with six rows of different sandwich bread to pick from, over eight brands, different types of grains, and different prices, the decision-making process could feel overwhelming without established preferences.

A big reason why we run into problems with self-esteem is that we forget we are not an object and don't need to sell our "self" to others to know we are loved and appreciated. We will spend time and money attempting to make our "self" into a desirable product believing that this is necessary to be valued. We will try to build and present an image of our "self" that will match peoples' value templates so they will want us.

Some of us get very skilled at doing this, motivated by safety reasons. I learned early on how to guess what others expected of me quite accurately and did my best to present that image for them to see. We come to believe we can control whether someone like us or not.

From this perspective, we come to believe that if we make our "self" valuable and desirable to someone, we will be given what we want: safety, time, attention, recognition, understanding, money, love, shelter, approval, etc. It's about exchanging value: I give you what you want that is important to you, in exchange for getting what is important to me, from you.

This is not right or wrong, but it can easily become a double-edged sword. When someone does NOT give us safety, time, attention, recognition, understanding, money, love or what we want, we come to believe they are not valuing us, and instead, are taking away our self-worth.

Looking at value this way means that when we don't get that promotion or recognition we wanted, we will feel devalued and unappreciated. Because our value was not affirmed and validated by getting the results we wanted, our self-esteem suffers. If our partner leaves us, withdrawing their love and attention, it will feel devaluing to us because we were deriving our sense of value from getting their love and attention. Now that these are gone, our self-esteem appears to have been lost.

Our "self" got interpreted to be an *object* whose value is dependent on its desirability and how well it meets the needs of others; as judged by their preference templates. If this *person-object* is discarded, passed up, left, rejected, etc. it will feel hurt because of its identification.

This hurt will only serve to reinforce the existing incorrect negative conclusions about our "self". It will feed the cycle that keeps us believing that we have to make our "self" into *some "thing"* valuable to others in order to get love, attention, recognition, or anything else we want or need. We have accepted the belief we are nothing without making our "self" into something valuable.

But let's pay attention to *what* gets hurt with disapproval, rejection, put-downs, etc. It is a "self" image that says, "I need someone's approval, acceptance, money, appreciation, attention, etc.", and needs reassurance that "I am not worthless or unwanted." When the self-image doesn't get that reassurance, we feel the emotional pain and suffering coming from our identification with this self-image. We then fearfully conclude, "It must be true. I am worthless."

Notice that it is not the rejection or disapproval per say that *causes* the hurt; it is our mind's negative *interpretation* and labeling of someone's response as "rejection" and "disapproval", believing this to be personal and feeling as if it says something bad about us. However, an underlying self-image that says "I am worthless" will already be present in our database and filtering the information in our situation so we interpret it as "rejection" and "disapproval". This is how the negative self-identity is proving itself true.

The fears around believing we are less than others can also put us into survival mode and can bring out the worst in us.

Let me demonstrate with a small example:

One day at the flea market a woven box caught my eye, so I approached the seller. I asked, "How much do want for the box?"

The woman said, "$20".

I liked the box, but for what I needed, the price was more than I was willing to pay.

So I asked, "What is the least you are willing to take?"

She said, "$20. I paid $36 for it new." She continued, "The difference between me and the other vendors is that I only sell quality items."

Something about her last statement made me want to argue with her. It triggered a reaction.

I wanted to challenge her and say, "Well, is that so? I just bought this quality mask for $3 from another vendor!" But I resisted this urge. I just said in a matter of fact way, "This is a flea market."

She said, "I have been coming here for six years and I know quality and what sells!"

I was not interested in her qualifications. I just needed a small, cheap, woven box.

I said, "I would be willing to give you $10, I don't need what is inside."

She quickly and indignantly replied, "No. It is a set! I also paid $7 for the paper grasshopper inside, and $10 is not even a fourth of what I paid all together!"

I paused because I noticed my heart pounding inside my chest. I immediately started to back away, but I kept my composure and calmly said, "This is not personal, either you want to sell it or not."

She replied quite irritated, "I don't see it that way! We just have different ways of seeing it!"

I agreed, and quickly left.

Later I recounted this event to my husband, feeling like I had been attacked for no reason. As I talked to him I was able to see that I had attacked the woman's judgment of value by devaluing her things (she was identified with her things) when I said, "This is a flea market." In other words, I doubted that her box was worth $20 there. This in turn was a defense reaction to what I had interpreted as a personal attack from her. In my mind, she had compared herself to the other vendors and judged herself *more than* by saying, "The difference between me and the other vendors is that *I only sell quality.*"

Some years back we had been vendors at that flea market. That alone was not the trigger that set me off, but I did identify my "self" as a "vendor". There was also an insecure self-image in my mind that said, "I am less than". Both my identification and my negative self-image interpreted the woman's comparison with the other vendors as saying, "I don't sell junk. I am better than the other sellers, including you."

This spurred a fight for self-importance and personal value. This was necessary because I was looking at my value as needing defense, believing she was trying to take it away. Here is the double edged sword again. If others can take my value away, then I must defend it and take it away from others to have more.

I could have decided to leave immediately after she said that the least she would be willing to take was $20. But did I see this as an option then? No. Her next sentence: "The difference between me and the other vendors is that I only sell quality items", triggered my identification with the pain of "I am less than". Now it felt like *she* had hurt *me* and so I had a right to defend my "self". It felt like my self-worth was at stake!

Someone else would not have interpreted her words the way I did. I overreacted. My sensitivity to her comment came from the fears that my negative belief was true. It is quite scary to believe that a person's value can be taken away and that some people can be *less than* and others *more than*. There was plenty of fear and hurt hiding here.

Unresolved fears and hurt will suck us into meaningless battles because it will feel like something personal is being taken away: our "self" respect, our honor, our importance, our spotlight, our dignity etc! This casual encounter turned into a fight for survival in my mind, and probably in hers too. The cause was my interpretation that feared I would be left without value if I let this woman believe she was "better than others, including me."

Did she really believe this? Who knows? The point is that even if she had believed it, beliefs are not Truth. I would have still been reacting to my interpretation, of her interpretation; of what she thought was true. My heart was not racing because of factual information, but from fear generated by my thoughts and perceptions.

Was my life or value ever in danger? No, but my interpretations made it seem that way, and I believed my interpretations to be truth. So, my body diligently followed without questioning this information, especially since my primitive survival mind was involved.

When we spend so much energy pursuing value or in battle for its protection, we are confirming the belief that we don't have enough of it. Competition and conflict become necessary to make sure we get our share. This identifies us with survival fears. This also supports the belief that self-esteem must be acquired from outside of us through our effort.

In the United States we tend to esteem, admire and look up to individuals that have distinguished their "self" and appear to stand above the crowd through their accomplishments. For example, people who achieve success despite difficult odds and who persevere despite their humble beginnings like the Horatio Alger story characters of the late 1800's, will tend to be highly regarded and esteemed.

There is a belief that individuals like these have *made something* of their "self" and so have *earned* high regard and admiration from others. We are comparing and measuring achievements, but since we identify with our achievements, it appears to us like these individuals have made their "self" worthy, and so we give them what they have *earned*, regard, praise and admiration.

Many of us have accepted the belief that it is possible to make our "self" worthy or unworthy, and we do it by earning it. In other words, we don't need to *take* away value from others because they will *give* it to us willingly; we just have to work hard to earn it. So, our achievements become very important to us.

It follows that having excelled in school, sports or the arts would give us the right to feel proud and worthy because others would agree that we have earned it. On the other hand, this often implies that we are not supposed to feel good about our "self" until we have earned it. If we haven't earned it, it can feel like we do not deserve nor have the right to feel worthy. From this perspective, achievement and the accompanying self-esteem serves to separate the worthy from the unworthy.

If we make achievement our strategy for gaining self-esteem, we can run into problems. Without claiming to always be number one in our field, how can our worth remain stable and sure? We would need to keep comparing our achievements constantly and need to be the best in all comparisons. Unfortunately, our self-esteem would become dependent on what and who we compare our achievements to.

I have a teenage son with a talent for music. However, he couldn't see this and in talking to him I found out why. He was comparing his playing, and himself, to the famous and professional guitar player, *Santana*. How could his playing measure up to someone with 50 years of professional guitar playing experience?

Who or what do you compare your "self" with? It is very possible that you are comparing as we say, "apples to oranges", like my son was. Perhaps you are not comparing your "self" to someone else but to an ideal self-image that is the standard for measuring your value. Trying to achieve a self-made ideal can often be more disheartening than measuring your "self" to someone else.

An ideal model can be so unrealistic that you can almost guarantee you will fall short. It can also be more difficult for you to feel good because it will be difficult to notice that you are making progress, since it won't come close to measuring up to the ideal. Not giving your "self" credit for the effort you are making can feel discouraging and will make it harder for you to keep going.

Our parents, schools, religions, media, society, culture, etc. teach us what is valuable in the world. They pass on their preference templates because that is what they have learned and believe is good, important and true. There is nothing bad about this. It has been going on for thousands of years. We all teach what we believe.

However, if we are struggling with self-esteem, we need to understand how our perceiving mind comes to its conclusions of worth to help us see our "self" in a better light. This will require letting go or revising many of our beliefs and values. I am not saying that what we have been taught does not have value. All I am saying is that it is important to examine our values and beliefs because, in the end, we are the ones living with the results and effects that come from them.

Chapter 14: Perfect Equality of the Self

As we saw in the previous chapter, self-esteem is dependent on comparison. Comparison is also dependent on perceiving differences. Without the perception of differences and inequality, the term self-esteem would be meaningless. If we saw no differences, we could not compare, nor distinguish any "self" from others. If we saw everyone as equal, there would be no basis for evaluation. This would not turn us into carbon copies of each other, but the surface difference that we have used to evaluate the worth of a person would not mean so much to us.

We notice differences like people's wealth, gender and skin color, among other things. In the history of Western World, society in general, has assigned more value to wealth than poverty; more to males than females; more to fair skin that dark skin; etc. Although we now understand that these are collective values, coming from subjective perceptions, nevertheless, for vast populations that are born into poverty and born female or a person of color, identification with such characteristics can still produce self-esteem issues.

This is not to say that white, wealthy males will not have self-esteem problems. I am just making the point that when someone is identified to a characteristic they are born with that is deemed less valuable by their society at large, their worth will appear to be tied to an apparent fact that they cannot easily change: the social economic status of their family, their gender and/or skin color.

This idea can be extended to other differences like sexual preference, religious affiliation, physical and mental handicaps, etc. One alternative to help bring more value to those identified with these characteristics would require bringing about social change in the preference templates of masses of people. You can see that the socially perceived value of women in the Western World has improved due to the efforts of the Feminist Movement. However, this approach requires concerted and collective effort and is slow. Perhaps there is another way?

I want to suggest to everyone, but in particular to those who have identified with one or more of these characteristics, that it is possible to change our perception and see beyond these differences.

But how can anyone deny differences based on facts like their economic status, color and gender? We do not need to deny anything. These facts, without the agreed upon social definitions of value we accepted, would be perceived by our mind as unimportant. This is why true change always begins within us and extends outward. So, it is possible to see beyond our differences to our fundamental equality and essential "Self".

Here is my example to demonstrate this point:

I lived in a small rural village in central Mexico for the first 7 years of my life. It was a subsistence farming community. I did not compare my "self" with others. Perhaps it was the age, or that we were all pretty much the same externally. I had no awareness of ethnicity, economic status and even gender since all my friends were girls, and I had little interaction with my brothers.

I had no notion of equality or inequality and therefore, could not give any meaning to such differences. They were not apparent. I wasn't physically blind to the differences, but without giving them meaning, it was like not seeing them. Remember that without existing beliefs, perception can easily miss things since there is no match.

But once we moved to California, I went to an Elementary School where no one spoke Spanish, and I did not speak one word of English. I became aware and saw the difference between me and the other kids. I became aware of my "ethnicity". I acquired a new identity that said "I am Mexican". By the end of First Grade I had concluded, "Mexicans are inferior to Anglo Americans."

From then on, I believed I would be seen as less than because of my ethnicity. I believed this because I accepted the label of "Mexican" as my identity. In my mind, "Mexicans" in comparison to "Anglo Americans" were different and not part of the norm. My child mind feared that differences determined status and value and that if someone was outside the norm of the majority (the ideal self-image), they were less than.

With regards to my gender identity, I was left without my girl friends when we moved. I began to interact more with my family, including three brothers living at home. As I began to mature, it was often pointed out that I was a girl, and I was supposed to take my place as such.

Interestingly enough, I did not accept this identity, or its unequal treatment. I saw no real reason why I should cook and clean for the boys, and I refused. I questioned the perception that being a girl made me different than boys. Feeling safe to assert my equality, I said "No." to both my mother and brothers who insisted I conform in belief and behavior to their perceptions. Thankfully, I had the full support of my father in standing up for my equality.

Again, it wasn't that I could not see I was a girl, the differences did not mean anything to me. As a result, I never identified my "self" with the label of "girl" nor with the social expectations and inferior value associated to the label. I did not make a self-image identity out of my gender.

However a couple years later, I accepted a deeply distorted identity based on our social-economic status. My intuition tells me that I already came in with this distorted view that said, "I am poor".

It took an event at age nine to bring it to my awareness:

My mother and I were at a second hand clothing store. I looked up and happened to see my mother slipping a small piece of clothing under her sweater. We left without paying for it. I was shocked! I judged her action shameful! Because I was identified with my family, I took on the shame. But in trying to explain what had taken place, knowing that my mother was a good person, I concluded that we had to be poor for her to resort to stealing.

From then on, I became very self-conscious of our economic situation and noticed differences in economic status everywhere. I was so embarrassed of where I lived; a converged two car garage with a patio extension, that once when my friend's mother gave me a car ride home, I told them I lived next door. I walked up to the neighbor's front door and waited for them to drive away before heading to my house.

You can clearly see how my self-esteem suffered believing that I was "less than" and "poor". My identification to these beliefs kept my attention focused on differences and inequality. How could I possibly see my full equality? But, when I refused to give meaning to my gender differences and did not accept a gender identity, my sense of worth and equality were not affected at all.

I can be 110% committed to the idea of equality now. But unless I can see my whole "self" as completely equal to others, despite surface differences, I will be supporting and contributing to the collective misperception of inequality in the external world. We must first see our fundamental "self" as equal, to have the world mirror back our perspective with social equality. Otherwise, our view will only be supporting stability in the external world's values and views of inequality.

There is a very deep Truth here. We are all essentially equal! It is not reflected perfectly in our external world because we are not seeing our complete equality within. When our perception is focused on comparing our "self" and seeing our differences, it is an indication that we are choosing to believe at some level, in the inequality of our "self" and others. Differences don't need to mean anything, unless we want to hold on to our perceiving mind's beliefs that are giving them meaning.

From working with older women clients who have struggled with low self-esteem and insecurity due to their gender identification, I see that healing requires letting go not just of society's definitions of value, but of our false self-image identities. We need to believe in the deeper Spiritual Truth of our being and its infinite and inherent value.

You may be thinking that I am asking for what appears to be a huge shift in "self" perception. Yet, I have certainty in my heart that it can be done. Connecting to the Truth that we are all fundamentally equal will release the idea of "self-esteem". If we understand and accept that everyone is truly equal, there is no need to compare or measure to ascertain our value. We can simply accept and appreciate our "self" just as we are, because we can see that we are NOT our physical characteristics or the current circumstances in our life.

In other words, true equality blinds us to judgments of value. The good news is that we are all just as worthy as the President of the United States. The President may still earn more money and have greater responsibility than us, but the worth of our being remains the same as his. How does that feel?

You may be wondering, "But how would the President feel?" Identify your "self" with the position of the President of the United States. Would it bother you to not be seen or treated in a "special" way due to your position?

Many of us would be bothered. Having others see and treat us more special is part of the reason why some of us strive to acquire high profile positions of influence in the first place. I want you to notice any resistance in your perceiving mind to true equality. True equality can be difficult to accept since it erases both the positive and negative scale of measurement.

If we don't want to be perceived as *less than*, we also need to accept not being perceived as *more than*. Accepting the truth of our equality means that no individual being is really better or worse, than another.

It may be easy to agree to let go of our negative "self" images and unworthiness, but equality also asks us to let go of the images that make us appear to be better than others. It is hard to give up not wanting to be better than others. This does not sit well with our egos. I know this well from personal experience.

Allow me to share:

I find myself getting ready to pay for my purchases at a large department store. I am amazed at how busy the store is today. I start walking to the fast lanes for 10 items or less, hoping those lines will be shorter than what I'm seeing. No luck. The two fast lanes are really long!

I notice a person walking in front of me also ready to pay. He lines up in one fast lane and I choose the other. I am feeling good as I compare the lines and think that I picked the shortest one and will beat this man to the cashier. As I wait, I am focused on how quickly the two lines are moving. Unfortunately, it appears that the other line is moving quicker.

I notice how my mind believes it is important that I get to the cashier first. I am not clear of the reason why this is important, but I start feeling a little anxious, so I begin EFT tapping (EFT is explained in more detail at the end of this book).

Discreetly I tap with my fingers on some acupuncture points on my face, hands and body, voicing my feelings in my mind:

"Even though getting to the cashier first is important to me; I deeply and completely accept myself. So, even though this feels like a competition and getting to the cashier first means that I'm smarter or better in some way; I deeply and completely accept myself. Even though I recognize that being first doesn't really make me better; there is an aspect (self-image) of me that really wants to distinguish itself and feel special; I deeply and completely accept myself."

I continue tapping expressing my feelings through my thoughts:

"It is important to be first; I need to win and feel like I am smarter because I picked the fastest line; I want to be more special than him; even though I recognize that I'm not really more special; an aspect (self-image) of me doesn't want to let this go; an aspect (self-image) of me wants to be special and doesn't want equality."

Aha! Here is a desire I had not been aware of before. I admit, sometimes being truthfully honest with my feelings uncovers desires and beliefs I'd rather deny. Nevertheless, getting to the buried information is always more important and good news despite any negative findings.

When I allow the negative beliefs to surface I can question them and let them go. In return, I receive greater understanding and compassion for my "self" and others. I can't begin to describe how rewarding this work is for me.

Here is what I discovered in my subconscious database this time:

I (identification with inequality) don't want equality because then I cannot be special, distinguished or better than somebody else. This aspect of my "self" must see itself as unimportant, since it goes to great extents to try to prove how special it is, through competition and comparison. It feels like equality would take away its drive to prove its "self" better that everyone else, and this is how it *gets* value. It feels like I (identification) need that drive! I (identification) am afraid that without that drive, I will languish in apathy, sit on my sofa all day and be a looser!

As I reflect on this experience, I come to the realization that there can never be complete equality as long as I hold on to my desire to be more special and better than others. I also realize that the self-image that wants to be more special has devised all sorts of structures in society and in my perceiving mind to prove that it is better than others. If it believed it was special or valuable enough, it would not be trying to prove this. It would already know its inherent worth with certainty.

Now I understood why I liked taking tests in school. To my kids this sounds strange. I saw each test as an opportunity to prove Mexicans were smart and good enough. Who was I trying to prove this to? Who really needed the convincing? My perceiving mind and its belief about my "self" that said, "Mexicans are inferior".

All self-images want to compete because this is how they accentuate differences and prove which is best. This is how they can feel reassured and know where they stand with respect to value and importance, but only in comparison to others. Also, self-images breed insecurity, uncertainty and sometimes havoc in our lives. Who wants that? I don't. I've had enough of self-images and their influence in my decisions and life.

Let me tell you why:

I was counseled in high school to major in engineering in college. I tried engineering, but after much soul searching and changes in major, I ended up studying and graduating with a degree in Sociology. Interestingly enough, I then applied to the MBA Program at Stanford University. I remember telling one of my friends, "If I get in, please remind me that I really don't want to go there." Yes, I admit this sounds crazy.

Let me explain. I knew that if I got in, I would judge myself insane to pass up the opportunity to go to the *number one* MBA program in the country. I was taught to value success and to climb as far as I could, if I could. But in my heart, I really didn't want to go there. I was asking my friend to help me because I had enough awareness to see that my thinking mind ruled over my heart. Deep down I knew I would be making a mistake if I got in and went.

So why did I even apply? I still needed to prove that I was not inferior, and getting in to this highly recognized and selective school was convincing. Did it matter that I did not really want to study business? No! My unconscious need to prove I was not inferior drove me to apply there so I could feel like I was *better than others*!

By the way, I did get in to the MBA program. My friend was no longer around to remind me I didn't want to go. I went. I studied one semester, took a year off, went back another semester and finally stopped going. I let go of needing to prove "Mexicans" are not inferior because the truth is, they are not inferior. We are all equal.

Beyond all self-images rests our true identity and our infinite worth. Our essential nature is unalterable because our being is not any *"thing"* that can be compared or that can perish or go out of style. Our being resides in the realm of Spirit beyond the physical level of existence and all perceptual understanding. It is the breath of Life manifesting though our Higher Mind and animating our body. It is what continues even when the body cannot.

Beyond all externals we can judge, is our essential nature: Spirit, Higher Self, Consciousness, God's Will, etc. However you want to label this deeper "Self", it is real. We have all experienced it at one time or another: in the breathless peace of a starry sky on a warm summer night; in the pure love of a sleeping newborn child; or in the enchantment and rapture of a beautiful song that touches our soul. It is in these moments when time disappears and for a second, everything is as it should be and is, good and pure, that we drink from the experience of just being.

Stripped of all images of "self" and false identities, we are as our Creator created us: divinely perfect in essence, completely equal and boundless in self-worth.

Chapter 15: The True Self

Perhaps you remember the children's book by P. D. Eastman called, *Are you my mother*? It is the story of a baby bird that hatches while his mother is away looking for worms. Since he does not see any other birds, he decides to go look for his mother. He stands on the edge of the nest and looks out for her. But he steps too far, and falls to the ground. Nevertheless, he is determined to find his mother and continues to look for her on foot.

Since he has no image of what his mother looks like, to every animal he meets along the way he asks, "Are you my mother? Each one responds with a "No.", some identifying themselves with their labels: I am a dog; I am a cow, etc. The little bird doesn't even know he is an animal. He sees an airplane up in the sky and yells, "Here I am, Mother."

This little bird reminds me of my own life's search for identity. Perhaps our story as humans is not that different from this little bird's. We spend our lives asking self-images to tell us what we are. All they can tell us is what we are NOT. It doesn't occur to us to look within. Instead, we venture away from the nest looking for our "self" not know who our Creator is, and all the time feeling lost and confused. From this perspective, it appears as if we were born a faceless nothing, without identity or value, without a mother, to reflect our inherent worth.

But life has a way of bringing us around full circle, just like the baby bird. The baby bird comes to a steam shovel and gets picked up and put back in its nest. When the mother bird returns with a worm, the baby bird says, "Yes, I know who you are... You are not a dog. You are not a cow. You are not a boat... You are a bird, and you are my mother." In seeing what he was NOT, the baby bird was able to recognize what he was and recognized his mother.

I hope I have helped you to see what you are NOT with this book. Much like this little bird, I spent much of my life looking to find my identity and self-worth, when it had never left me, in Truth.

We are as we were created. We are children of the Source of Life. Our perceiving mind cannot comprehend this

Truth, but our Higher Mind can resonate to it. We have human form but our essential being resides at the Spirit level. We can only be a part of that which created us.

We all share equally of Life. When we recognize "our mother", Creator, we come to know our identity with certainty because we cannot be different. That is why our true identity and our worth are unbounded, beyond measurement, belief and change.

Our inherent value and self-esteem is beyond our perception, but not beyond our recognition. From the place within all of us that holds wisdom and Truth, comes the certainty that our worth is unbounded and therefore, immeasurable. There is no point in comparing our "self". Our worth cannot fluctuate or be changed in Truth. Letting go of our misperceptions will help us reclaim this Truth.

We all have the Light of Truth within. Choose to see your "self" in that pure Light. In doing so, your perception will eventually come to see the biggest secret you have been hiding from your "self"; that you are one with the Light!

"What you are is not established by your perception, and is not influenced by it at all. Perceived problems in identification at any level are not problems of fact. They are problems of understanding, since their presence implies a belief that what you are is up to you to decide." *The Course in Miracles Text* (Pg. 125, Chap. VI, Section 9, Verses 3-5).

In our lifetime, we are not deciding what we are, but what we want to believe we are. You can keep wanting to believe you are your "self" images and what you *make* or *fail to make* of your "self"; giving your perceiving mind the power to determine your worth and value. Or, you can choose to believe that your Identity has already been established with immeasurable worth unalterable by the judgments of your perceiving mind.

Choose to align the perceptions of your "self" with all that is positive and good. In this manner, you can come to see your "self" in a positive light, but more importantly, come to recognize your Identity as part of the One Light that shines through all consciousness!

Chapter 16: Emotional Freedom Techniques (EFT)

EFT (Emotional Freedom Techniques) or EFT tapping is an emotional version of acupuncture except without the use of needles. Instead, you stimulate key acupuncture points on your head, face and body by tapping on them with your fingertips.

The mechanical process is easy to memorize and can be done anywhere. Of course, there is more to EFT tapping than just the physical tapping sequence. We are working with attention and intention. We are learning to stay present in the moment while we focus our attention on the issue or emotion we are working to release. Our intention is to find the Truth that heals the hurt.

The combination of the physical tapping, the emotional connection and the observing presence of our Higher Mind, unblocks stuck energy showing up as negative emotions and beliefs, releasing them from our energy system. This helps shift the interpretations of our past negative experiences, allowing us to let go of any negative beliefs and judgments supported by those events. By releasing the intensity associated with what shows up in our conscious awareness as we tap, we are releasing the energy that anchors trauma, negative beliefs and self images into our database and keep us feeling stuck.

Great technical skill is not involved. What is necessary is being present while we turn our attention inward, observing with honesty and courage the perceiving mind's world of emotions, memories and beliefs. It is a journey of excavating old, non-serving thought patterns, reactions and self-made images to revise or let them go.

From my perspective, EFT is a tool that can help us find the truth of our identity, one that our perceiving mind often resists.

EFT Tapping History:

In 1980, Dr. Callahan discovered quite by accident the beginning of what he later called, TFT (Thought Field Therapy). He had been trying to help a client clear an intense water phobia with traditional therapy without success. He happened to be sitting with his client a few yards away from a swimming pool one day, when it occurred to him to have her tap under her eye with her fingertips. He was remembering that this point fell on the stomach acupuncture meridian. To his great amazement, the client jumped out of her chair and ran towards the pool, no longer afraid of the water. Her phobia never returned.

Emotional Freedom Techniques was made available to therapist in 1995. Gary Craig developed it after having been trained by Dr. Roger Callahan in Thought Field Therapy. Gary emphasizes:

"I am neither a psychologist nor a licensed therapist. Rather, I am a Stanford engineering graduate and an ordained minister and, although we don't pound the table for God here, I do come at this procedure from a decidedly spiritual perspective. My ordained ministry is with the Universal Church of God in Southern California which is non-denominational and embraces all religions. I am an avid student of A Course In Miracles but at no time is any EFT'er asked to follow any specific spiritual teaching. I was born April 13, 1940 and have been intensely interested in personal improvement via psychology since age 13. That was when I recognized that the quality of my thoughts was mirrored in the quality of my life. Since then I have been self taught in this field, seeking only those procedures that, in my opinion, produced results. EFT is my latest finding, the core of which I learned from Dr. Roger Callahan. I also have high regard for Neuro Linguistic Programming (NLP) in which I am a Certified Master Practitioner."

Gary Craig modified the TFT techniques and introduced EFT to the world in 1999 by making the EFT Handbook and the EFT Library Training Videos available via the internet. This is how I was introduced to EFT, later receiving my EFT Certifications.

The great contribution that Gary has made to what he called the "Healing High Rise", is not yet widely recognized or appreciated by the general public, but I am positive it will be in the future. My deep gratitude goes to him and his work of love.

For more information on EFT, how it works and about my EFT Practice visit: www.healing-with-eft.com

Did you find this book interesting, helpful or worth your reading, or not? Please take a couple of minutes to leave me your sincere book review below:

http://www.amazon.com/Beyond-Self-Esteem-Discovering-Self-Worth-
ebook/dp/B0082ZYR7C/ref=sr_1_2?ie=UTF8&qid=1350494101&sr=8
-2&keywords=Beyond+self-
esteem%3A+Discovering+Your+Boundless+Self-worth

. Thank you and blessings!

Made in the USA
San Bernardino, CA
09 April 2017